C000049221

VITAMIN DEFICIENCY

Causes & Prevention

by Dr Leonard Mervyn

BSc, PhD, C.Chem, FRSC

Amberwood Publishing Ltd
Park Corner, Park Horsley, East Horsley, Surrey KT24 5RZ
Telephone: 01483 285919

© Amberwood Publishing Ltd 1995

First Edition 1995

All rights reserved. No part of this publication may be reproduced,
stored in a retrievable system or transmitted in any form or by any means
electronic, mechanical, photocopying, recorded or otherwise without
prior permission from the publishers Amberwood Publishing Ltd.

© Authors Copyright Dr Leonard Mervyn 1995

ISBN 1-899308-11-3

Cover design by Design Hive

Typeset and designed by
Word Perfect, Christchurch, Dorset.

Printed in Great Britain

CONTENTS

Note to Reader

Whilst the author has made every effort to ensure that the contents of this book are accurate in every particular, it is not intended to be regarded as a substitute for professional medical advice under treatment. The reader is urged to give careful consideration to any difficulties which he or she is experiencing with their own health and to consult their General Practitioner if uncertain as to its cause or nature. Neither the author nor the publisher can accept any legal responsibility for any health problem which results from use of the self-help methods described.

About the Author

Dr. Leonard Mervyn is a Clinical Biochemist, experienced in pharmaceutical research and with a special interest in Vitamins and Minerals. He was the first to discover Coenzyme Q10 in man and identified the active form of vitamin B12, methylcobalamin, in human blood. He has written many books and scientific papers and has been honoured both by a Cressy Morrison Award from the New York Academy of Sciences and by an Italseber Gold Medal from the University of Pavia. He is currently the Technical Director of a major Healthcare Company, and is both a fellow of The Royal Society of Chemistry and The Royal Society of Health. In addition to his other interests, Dr. Mervyn is an external examiner for Oxford University.

1 | Introduction

The term vitamin is attributed to the Polish chemist Casimir Funk who coined it from "vita" (meaning life), and "amine" (a class of chemical substances to which vitamins were assigned, albeit incorrectly). Funk merely put a name to a concept of micronutrients, usually present in food, that are essential to maintain health in animals and man. This idea was originally suggested by the British biochemist, Sir Frederick Gowland Hopkins.

Strictly speaking, a true vitamin should satisfy certain criteria before being acceptable as such, and these are:

1 They are needed only in small amounts.
2 Adequate amounts should be supplied in the diet.
3 When they are deficient the individual shows distinct clinical symptoms and disease.
4 That disease and these symptoms are cured only by treatment with that specific vitamin.

As we shall see, these are only generalizations since there are exceptions to every criterion. For example, certain fats and amino acids (from proteins) are essential for health and can only be obtained from the diet, but the relatively large quantities needed puts them outside the first criterion, although they satisfy the other three. Some vitamins are made within the body, either in the tissues themselves or by bacteria that inhabit the intestine, but it is debatable whether sufficient for the body's needs can be met in this way. A deficiency of a single vitamin of the vitamin B complex is rare so symptoms may be related to lack of more than one. Similarly, treatment to overcome these symptoms may require multivitamin therapy, although in specific cases only one vitamin need be given.

In the early days of vitamin research, vitamins were conveniently put into one of two categories, namely, fat-soluble and water-soluble. Although this separated them on the basis of their physical property, later studies indicated the two types were also different in their functions within the body. We shall see later what these are, but let us first look at the vitamins we know exist.

The fat-soluble vitamins are designated A, D, E and K. There is also beta-carotene known as a provitamin because the body can convert it to vitamin A. Although this is an important source of the vitamin in vegetarians and vegans because they are not eating pre-formed vitamin A found only in foods of animal, fish and poultry origins, beta-carotene has important functions in its own right. These include its protective function in the body as an antioxidant, as are vitamins C and E. Certain *polyunsaturated fatty acids* were once known as Vitamin F but this designation is falling into disuse to be replaced by the term *EFA* or *Essential Fatty Acids*. The required daily intake of EFA is measured in grams which rather puts them outside the province of true vitamins despite their being necessary for health.

The water-soluble vitamins consist of the members of the vitamin B complex and vitamin C. The vitamin B complex consists of eight, eleven or thirteen members, depending upon which authority you believe. For the purpose of this book we shall regard the true vitamin B complex as a mixture of *eight* different substances. The other possible members are still in contention but we shall consider their possible therapeutic uses later.

The eight true vitamins in the B complex are thiamine (vitamin B1), *riboflavine* (vitamin B2), *niacin* (vitamin B3), *pantothenic acid* (vitamin B5), *pyridoxine* (vitamin B6), *cobalamin* (vitamin B12), *folic acid and biotin.* The three members loosely associated with the complex are *choline, inositol* and *para-aminobenzoic acid (PABA)*. You will see that the trivial names are given first with the appropriate number in parentheses. This is because there is now an increasing tendency to characterise vitamins by name in the regulations laid down by various authorities so as to avoid past ambiguities in the numbering of the members of the vitamin B complex.

One reason why the first eight members of the vitamin B complex fall neatly into one category is because they all function in a similar manner. To explain this we must look at the fundamental principle of life itself.

All forms of life, ranging from the simple one-cell organisms, like yeasts or bacteria, to the highly complex human being, are based on a mass of biochemical reactions. Life itself depends upon these chemical changes which regulate the way we digest food and break it down into simpler components; the way these nutrients are turned into energy; the way this energy translates into the movement of life; the way the biochemicals in food enable the brain and nervous system to function; the way essential nutrients are built up into new blood, flesh and other tissues. These biochemical reactions actually determine the processes upon which life is sustained. However, they cannot occur at a rate to sustain life without a catalyst to speed up these processes.

Substances that produce chemical change in the body, and indeed in any living thing, are known as *enzymes*. They are sometimes referred to as *organic catalysts* or *accelerators*, but whatever the name, the function is the same, to quicken life's processes. Enzymes are all specific types of *proteins* and we rely upon the body to produce its own supply of them. Unfortunately, most of these enzymes cannot function alone as they require some other factors to help them perform their roles. These factors are known as *coenzymes*, and these in turn are *vitamins*, usually those of the vitamin B complex.

It is easy to see, therefore, how important vitamins are to the processes of life. Without vitamins, life-sustaining reactions slow down because the enzymes cannot function without their coenzymes. Symptoms of ill-health will follow and eventually death may result. Adequate intakes of the B vitamins are hence necessary on a regular basis to ensure body levels are maintained at a suitable level. Fortunately, enzymes and coenzymes (vitamins) are not destroyed when they are performing their life-giving functions and are used over and over again. However, some losses, due mainly to excretion of vitamins, are inevitable, so without a constant dietary intake a slow, insidious deficiency will result.

Although much is known about the functions of the vitamin B complex as coenzymes, the other vitamins appear to work in other ways. Vitamins C and E, for example, have important protective roles within the body; vitamin C in the fluid of the organs and vitamin E in the fatty tissues. Vitamin K has one unique function, that of ensuring the clotting capacity of the blood is maintained. Vitamin A supports a healthy skin, mucous (wet) membranes and eyes, as well as performing a unique role in the process of sight. Vitamin D is solely concerned with ensuring efficient absorption of calcium and phosphorus from the diet. In none of their functions do these vitamins appear to act as coenzymes but rather directly or indirectly as essential substances in their own right.

When we look at our minimum needs of these essential vitamins on a daily basis the surprising thing to emerge is the vast variation in their quantities required. At the two extremes are vitamin C at about 100 milligrams (one three-hundredth of an ounce), or one-tenth of one gram, and vitamin B12 at one microgram, or one millionth of one gram. The others fall somewhere in between. These differences may reflect the proportionate amounts present in the food and probably represent how man has aligned to his diet over the millions of years of evolution. What is highly significant is that the inability to absorb just one-millionth of one gram of vitamin B12 daily leads to just as grave consequences as does the lack of the other vitamins needed in much larger amounts. All are important for health – none can replace another.

A note on vitamin measurement

You may come across vitamins expressed as international units (i.u.) as well as or instead of weight (milligrams or micrograms). International units are a left-over from the days of vitamin research when the chemical structures of the micronutrients were unknown and scientists measured them in terms of biological activity, i.e. their effect upon some physiological function of an animal. Later as they were isolated and as their structures became known, vitamins could be measured in terms of their weight and international units became obsolete. Nevertheless, some have persisted and, today, vitamins A, D and E may be expressed in international units on labels. The relationships are as follows:

VITAMIN A   1 microgram = 3.33 i.u.
VITAMIN D   1 microgram = 40 i.u.
VITAMIN E   1 milligram = 1 i.u. dl-alpha tocopheryl acetate
VITAMIN E   1 milligram = 1.36 i.u. d-alpha tocopheryl acetate
VITAMIN E   1 milligram = 1.1 i.u. dl-alpha tocopherol
VITAMIN E   1 milligram = 1.49 i.u. d-alpha tocopherol
VITAMIN E   1 milligram = 0.89 i.u. dl-alpha tocopherol succinate
VITAMIN E   1 milligram = 1.21 i.u. d-alpha tocopherol succinate

Note

1 gram (g) = 1000 milligrams (mg)
1 milligram (mg) = 1000 milligrams (μg)
1 kilogram (kg) = 1000 grams (g)

2 | How our diet is robbed of vitamins

Having established that our food as provided by nature contains all the vitamins we need for health, let us look now how those vitamins can be depleted by the way we treat our food from the time it is picked or butchered, to when it is eaten.

Storage and processing

Simply storing vegetables can give rise to serious losses of vitamin C. Potatoes, for example, when freshly dug from the ground will contain about 30mg of vitamin C per 100g (3.5oz). After three months storage, in the dark and at ordinary temperatures, this level has dropped to 20mg per 100g; after five months it is only 15mg per 100g; after seven months it is reduced to 10mg per 100g; after nine months only 8mg vitamin C is left in 100g potatoes. To many people potatoes represent the main source of their daily vitamin C intake and when these are old, as in the spring months before the new crops appear their contribution of vitamin C is minimal. This is the reason why some old people, particularly in low income groups and where fruit is perceived as expensive, develop symptoms of abject scurvy during the month of April. Once the new potatoes appear and are eaten they contain enough vitamin C to cure the condition until months later when, after the vitamin has been depleted in the stored vegetables, the deficiency cycle starts again.

Even storage of foods at refrigeration, or freezer temperatures, can lead to substantial losses. Vitamin E is lost readily at deep freeze temperatures of $-12°C$. Potato crisps, for example, which can supply useful amounts of the vitamin from the vegetable oil in which they are cooked (although they are generally thought to be of low nutritional value and are usually termed junk food), will lose 68 percent and 74 percent of their vitamin E after storage at $-12°C$ for periods of one month and two months respectively. The B vitamin pantothenic acid disappears slowly from all types of food that are kept frozen.

Air and light are the greatest natural destroyers of vitamins. Riboflavin is readily converted into a compound called lumiflavin by the action of light. Unfortunately, lumiflavin in turn destroys vitamin C. Hence, if milk is left for long periods in sunlight or even under shop lights not only does the riboflavin disappear but vitamin C losses are also substantial.

Milk remains one of our more important sources of riboflavin so such losses can be serious. Milk should, therefore, be transferred to a refrigerator as soon as possible after delivery or collection to preserve its vitamin content. Other vitamins that are readily broken down by light include A, carotene and B12.

Some vitamins are readily oxidised and hence destroyed by the action of the oxygen in the air. Whilst many storage conditions exclude air, it is easy to inadvertently destroy vitamin C, for example, by commonplace practices. Fruit juices and drinks are often taken for their vitamin C content but this can be reduced rapidly once the container has been opened. Studies have indicated that orange drink preparations lost between 30 and 50 percent of their vitamin content within eight days of opening a sealed bottle; after three to four weeks 90 percent had been lost. Losses were accelerated by shaking the bottles vigorously – a practice that is common amongst consumers. The vitamin C in apple juice is lost even more rapidly. 50 percent was lost after four days; 95 percent was destroyed after only 16 days storage at the relatively low temperature of 5°C, which is lower than the average domestic refrigerator. Fruit and vegetable juices are a pleasant and convenient way of taking vitamin C, but there is little to be gained by storing them for long periods once the container is opened. Careful decanting from the container will also help to preserve the vitamin from the destructive action of air.

All fruit and vegetables lose vitamins when stored at ambient temperatures. Some are preserved to a large extent by storing at deep freeze temperatures and this must be regarded as the best way to retain food for long periods. Do not forget however that before freezing, vegetables are blanched and this process can contribute to losses of vitamins even before the food is frozen. The best way to maintain the vitamin potency of food is to eat it as fresh as possible and avoid long periods of storage. If it must be stored, keep it at deep freeze temperatures.

The drying of some foods can also adversely affect certain vitamins. Dried vegetables and fruits lose virtually all of their vitamin C during the drying process but the B vitamins at least survive in the main. Freeze-drying represents the least destructive method of removing water but for most foods this process has not yet reached commercial levels.

Carotene losses in vegetables and fruits range from 10-20 percent under controlled, mild conditions of drying to virtually complete destruction in traditional open-air drying. Storage losses of both vitamin A and carotene can be substantial in certain foods even at refrigerator temperatures.

Butter loses up to 30 percent of its vitamin A content after twelve months at 5°C; at higher room temperatures (as in the tropics) losses are 35 percent after only five months. For some reason, vitamin A and carotene are far more stable in margarines – possibly because of the differing fatty acid contents. Similarly, destruction of vitamin A is minimal in skimmed milk powder after three months even at blood temperatures but serious losses occur after twelve months.

The critical time for both vegetable foods and those of animal origin appears to be about three months. It is only after this time that losses start to become significant. Hence any storage beyond this time can seriously affect the vitamin A and carotene contents of all foods. Remember that these periods are measured from the time of manufacture so that when the foods reach your refrigerator their shelf life could already have been some weeks. The existence of 'butter mountains' in the EEC community and the relatively slow turnover of this foodstuff is likely to render the product virtually devoid of these vitamins once it reaches the consumer.

Don't imagine that all the vitamins in raw foodstuffs start disappearing once the food has left the ground or the tree because vitamins vary widely in their stability. Vitamins B2, C and E are particularly susceptible in this respect but the remainder of the vitamin B complex will still be there when the food is eaten or cooked. Bruising of vegetables and fruits is particularly harmful to these unstable vitamins because it breaks down cells within the structure of the fruit and vegetable. Enzymes are released and these can have a destructive effect upon the micronutrients. Within the intact cell everything is kept in order and separated by intercell partitioning so there is no chance of interaction. Once cell walls are broken the contents mix and the introduction of air accelerates destruction of the vitamins. Intact food substances have a stabilising effect upon vitamins as they protect them from light and air. It is only bad handling and storage, combined with destructive cooking methods, which bring about a decline in the level of vitamins present in food.

The refining and processing of basic foodstuffs can also contribute to loss and destruction of some vitamins. For an example we need look no further than the refining of wholemeal flour to the popular white variety. All the vitamins present in wholemeal or wholewheat flour are reduced drastically when refined into white flour. These losses are so serious that government legislation forces millers to put back thiamine and nicotinic acid into white flour. Even with this fortification, however, the levels of thiamine and nicotinic acid in white flour are 32.6 percent and 64.3 percent lower respectively than in the wholemeal type. Unfortunately, the drastic reductions in other vitamins content that result from the refining of flour are not redressed so white flour and the products made from it are grossly depleted of vitamins.

Similar losses of vitamins are encountered when raw cane sugar is converted into the pure white variety. Hence what is a useful food with its full complement of vitamins and minerals as supplied by nature becomes simply a source of calories only – an 'empty calorie' food. Rice too is virtually depleted of its vitamins when it is refined from the raw, unpolished natural variety into the more popular but less nutritious white rice. Dried potato products often have added vitamin C but this is only a replacement for the natural material destroyed during the drying process.

Fat soluble vitamins too are lost by food refining – the vitamin E in wholegrain wheat is neatly disposed of during the production of white flour. Serious losses also occur when cooking oils are extracted from grains, seeds and beans since vitamin E does not stand up to the solvents and heating applied during their extraction. Vitamin A, and Carotene particularly, do survive most refining processes as long as light is excluded.

The reasons why refining certain wholefoods causes wholesale loss of vitamins are twofold. First, as in the case of grains and rice, the portion disposed of, like the bran, is the main source of vitamins and of minerals. Second, the methods used in refining are often destructive because of the applications of heat and solvents, etc. At least in the first case the vitamins can be reclaimed by utilizing the part removed, like the bran or wheatgerm. In the second case they are lost forever.

The losses we have discussed above have usually occurred before the food has reached our kitchens. Let us now look at how cooking processes can also contribute to a depletion of vitamins. In addition, we shall see how a little thought and trouble can retain these essential micronutrients during the cooking of food, at least when under our control in the kitchen.

How vitamins are lost in cooking

Most of the food we eat is cooked, either by ourselves in the kitchen, or in a factory by a food manufacturer, or in a take-away fast food supplier. The act of cooking itself can cause losses of vitamins from that food but there are distinct differences in how we can control those losses. In the kitchen, cooking losses can be regained to a large extent; when the food is prepared elsewhere the lost vitamins are gone forever. Food losses of vitamins during cooking processes are a combination of partial destruction of these sensitive micronutrients and those amounts that are leached out into the cooking fluids. We can limit the actual destruction of vitamins but can't do much about them once they are gone. Leached vitamins can be recovered. Fortunately, in most domestic cooking processes, the losses due to leaching far outweigh the quantities irreversibly destroyed. The factors that determine the extent of cooking losses of vitamins during cooking are:

1. The method of cooking.
2. The time of cooking.
3. The temperature of cooking.
4. The volume of water or of cooking fat in which the food is cooked.
5. The physical state of the food being cooked.

In boiling vegetables, for example, the highest losses are associated with a large volume of boiling water, a prolonged boiling time, and finely divided vegetables. Both carotene and vitamin E, because they are fat-soluble, are not affected by the boiling process, irrespective of whether the vegetable is the root kind, the leafy type or is a seed, e.g. peas, beans. All the watersoluble vitamins, i.e. the vitamin B complex and C, are lost to a certain extent when these types of vegetables are boiled, usually between 30 and 50 percent of the original content. Fortunately, most of these losses are simply leaching into the boiling water so they can be recovered by utilizing that water.

VITAMIN C

This is the most unstable of the vitamins and its losses during cooking processes can be quite substantial.

The proportion of losses due to destruction and those due to leaching is from 10 percent to 55 percent and from less than 10 percent to 60 percent respectively. Steaming and pressure cooking of green vegetables and of root vegetables destroy from 20 to 40 percent of the vitamin C present but the percentage lost by leaching is less than 10 percent. The reverse occurs in simple boiling of these vegetables.

The other water-soluble vitamins behave in a similar fashion. If the cooking water is utilized in some way, the percentage of vitamin C available to the body increases to 60-90 in all cases.

These figures apply only to a once-cooked vegetable. If this is stored then re-heated at a later date, losses are much more substantial and in some cases virtually all the vitamin is destroyed. There is a classic case on record of a children's hospital in Vienna where 40 out of 64 children who were long-stay patients, developed scurvy because of the practice of feeding them re-heated vegetables. These vegetables were boiled in bulk for long periods; the water was discarded; the boiled vegetables were set aside and re-heated at daily intervals. Little wonder that their vitamin C content turned out to be virtually zero!

Beware, too, of another common practice, especially where large quantities of foods are prepared in advance. Potatoes and other root vegetables when soaked overnight in cold water will lose up to 60 percent of their vitamin C content by leaching into the water. If the water is discarded most of the original vitamin C will accompany it down the drain. Similarly, machine peeling of vegetables is more destructive to the vitamin C than the hand process. This then is another practice associated with large scale, institutional preparation of foods that leads to wholesale losses of vitamin C and the other water-soluble vitamins.

Not surprisingly, the large-leafed vegetables, like cabbage, which present a high surface area to the boiling water are the more likely to lose their vitamin C by leaching. Boiling cabbage for 20 minutes reduced its vitamin C content by 70 percent; simmering it at 70 to 80°C for 60 minutes reduced it by 90 percent. Fortunately, the vitamin can be recovered in the main by using the water to make a sauce, or gravy, or in some other way.

Root vegetables, like potatoes, will lose more vitamin C if they are diced than if they are cooked whole. The following losses in potatoes are those expected with the appropriate cooking technique mentioned; peeled, boiled then mashed 30 to 50 percent; unpeeled boiled 20 to 40 percent; baked 20 to 40 percent; roast 20 to 40 percent; steamed 20 to 40 percent; chipped 25 to 35 percent lost. This means that new potatoes subjected to these methods will supply between 18 and 24mg vitamin C per 100g (3.5 oz.) as eaten. When the potatoes are old, they will provide only between 4.8 and 6.4mg vitamin C per 100g. This is not sufficient to supply even the minimum daily quantity needed to prevent the deficiency disease scurvy.

The B Vitamins

THIAMINE

Amongst the B vitamins, thiamine (vitamin B1) is the least stable which may explain why, according to the World Health Organisation, this vitamin is the one most likely to be deficient in diets worldwide. It is stable only under acid conditions, which means that any alkaline treatment of foods containing the vitamin will destroy most of it. Trace minerals, like copper, present in some cooking utensils, will accelerate the destruction of thiamine. Sulphur dioxide, widely used to preserve foodstuffs, completely inactivates the vitamin.

This preservative is often added to mince both to prolong the shelf-life of the meat and to maintain its attractive red colour. Forty-eight hours after treating mince with sulphur dioxide, the thiamine content is reduced by 90 percent. You should therefore avoid sulphur dioxide treated meats if you wish to preserve your intake of thiamine. Similarly, beware of ready-peeled potatoes which are kept white by adding sulphite solution (i.e. sulphur dioxide in water). This treatment will dispose of about 55 percent of the thiamine originally present in the potatoes. As these vegetables are the only ones that contribute significant quantities of thiamine to the diet, using preserved or commercially processed potatoes as the main source of the vegetable, will add insignificant amounts of the vitamin and lead to the development of deficiency.

Although you must be aware of losses of thiamine in cooking processes, in good quality foods the protein and amino acids present will help protect the vitamin. Starches also assist in the absorption of thiamine. This is why cereals, which contain both protein and starch, are added to tinned meats, particularly those containing pork which represents a very rich source of thiamine. Cereals are thus excellent natural preservatives of the thiamine in cooked meats.

Apart from destruction of the vitamin by processing methods often carried out before you buy the food, the principal losses of thiamine are due to its water solubility. The more finely divided or ground the food is, the greater the loss. Chopped and minced foods can lose from 20 to 70 percent of their thiamine but it can be recovered by eating the extracted liquors. When meat is cooked at 150°C there is virtually no destruction of the vitamin but there are considerable losses into the exuded juices, although these can be recovered of course. At temperatures of 200°C however, at least 20 percent of the thiamine is destroyed. Over-cooking of meat should therefore be avoided if you wish to preserve its thiamine content.

The instability of thiamine in alkaline substances is illustrated nicely by observing its losses from boiled rice. When pure, distilled water is used, losses are nil. Tap water which is slightly alkaline causes 8 to 10 percent loss; the more alkaline well water gives rise to 36 percent loss.

Simple baking processes cause 15 to 25 percent destruction of thiamine, but when baking powder is added (this is highly alkaline) at least half the vitamin is destroyed.

When bread is baked, between 15 and 30 percent of the thiamine content of the flour is destroyed. Most of the destruction takes place in the crust so the popular practice of removing this part of the bread before eating it is not laying one open to B1 deficiency. Remember, that further losses of thiamine will result when the bread is toasted. Light toast is to be preferred to the darker variety if you wish to minimise thiamine losses.

Meats represent a very important source of thiamine in the diet so losses encountered in the various ways of cooking it can vary from 30 to 80 percent with roasting and braising being the least destructive processes. Remember, however, to utilize the various juices that are produced during these cooking methods if you want to ensure the maximum intake of thiamine. If the meat you cook has been frozen, be sure to utilize the liquids dripped during the thawing — these are rich sources of leached vitamin B 1. In the canned variety, use of the juices.

Thiamine losses from fish also depend upon the cooking method used, e.g. percentage losses are poaching, 10; baking, 30; frying, 40; grilling, 20. In some countries, notably Japan, raw fish represents an important item of food but when eaten uncooked, thiamine can be lost. The reason is that raw fish contains an enzyme called thiaminase which destroys thiamine whilst the food is in the gastro-intestinal system. Normal cooking methods will destroy thiaminase but this of course survives if the fish is eaten raw. There are many cases on record of thiamine deficiency, sometimes leading to beriberi, in Japanese who eat large amounts of raw fish.

Losses of thiamine during the cooking of vegetables depends largely on the type of vegetable. Root vegetables will lose 25 percent; leafy vegetables will lose 40 percent; seeds lose 30 percent. Milk is a useful source of thiamine but losses can occur during the various processing methods as the following percentage losses show: pasteurization 10; sterilisation 20; UHT 10; boiling 0.

RIBOFLAVIN

The vitamin (also known as B2) is stable to air, acid and heat up to 130°C. The most destructive elements are alkalis and light. Because of its water solubility, riboflavin is readily lost by leaching from chopped foods in wet processing and cooking methods.

Light must be excluded if the riboflavin in foodstuffs is to be preserved, particularly in liquid foods like milk. Even a relatively low level of destruction of riboflavin to the product lumiflavin (5 percent) can cause 50 percent of the vitamin C content to be destroyed by the action of the lumiflavin. Studies indicate that milk exposed to light in summer loses 90 percent of its riboflavin content in full sunshine in 2 hours; 45 percent in cloudy weather; 30 percent when the sky is completely clouded over. Room lighting causes 30 percent loss within 24 hours. Bread, too, is affected by light. Supermarket lighting destroyed 17 percent of the riboflavin content of bread rolls in 24 hours; 13 percent when the rolls were wrapped in amber plastic film; 2 percent when wrapped in orange plastic.

Although riboflavin is perfectly stable in cold storage beef when light is excluded, losses can occur once it is cooked. 20 percent is lost during the roasting, frying and grilling of meats and poultry; 30 percent is lost when meat and poultry is stewed or boiled. Similarly, whilst the vitamin is stable in raw, fresh fish, percentage losses during the following cooking processes are: poaching 0; baking 20; frying or grilling 20. When vegetables are cooked percentage losses of riboflavin are 30 (root-type); 40 (leafy-type); 30 (seed-type). When possible, therefore, it is wise to eat vegetables raw to ensure the maximum intake of riboflavin. When this is not possible, as for example in certain seeds and pulses, the losses induced by cooking can be counteracted by eating the cooking fluids.

Milk and meats represent our most important sources of dietary riboflavin. Cold milk that has had the minimum exposure to light is an excellent food in this respect but boiling it will reduce the riboflavin content by between 12 and 25 percent. Pasteurized milk will have lost about 14 percent of its riboflavin content when it reaches you but the rest of the vitamin can be preserved by taking the precautions in storing mentioned above. Dry or wet curing of meats will cause 40 percent loss in riboflavin level so this should be taken into account and regarded as additional to further losses induced by various cooking methods.

NICOTINIC ACID

This is the most stable of the B complex of vitamins so losses in cooking are mainly a result of leaching. The vitamin is unaffected by heat, air, light, acidity, alkalinity and by sulphite or sulphur dioxide. There are losses of 20 percent of the nicotinic acid content of meats and poultry when they are roasted, fried or grilled; and of 50 percent when these foodstuffs are stewed or boiled. Fish will lose 10 percent when poached and 20 percent when baked, fried or grilled. Root vegetables and seeds will lose 30 percent of their nicotinic acid content when boiled; leafy vegetables will lose 40 percent. All of these losses can be recovered and made available to the diet simply by utilizing the cooking water of juices. Remember too, that some will be lost into the thawed drippings, from frozen foods but these also are recoverable.

Nicotinic acid is unique amongst the vitamins in that it can be liberated from certain foods by the cooking process. This is because in cereals the vitamin is bound to starches and proteins in a complex called niacytin. This complex is resistant to digestion by the normal digestive processes of the body. In wheat flour, a significant 77 percent of its nicotinic acid content is present in this bound form. The best way to liberate the free nicotinic acid is to bake the flour with alkaline baking powder. In Mexico, maize (corn) is soaked overnight in lime water before using it to make the staple food tortillas. This practice makes the nicotinic acid content of maize available in the diet. It was a prime factor in ensuring that Mexican peasants did not suffer from nicotinic acid deficiency (a disease called "Pellagra") in the 1920's, when their USA counterparts over the border were dying from pellagra because their cooking techniques with the same raw food ingredients did not liberate the vitamin.

All the processing techniques used in milk and milk products and those utilizing eggs do not affect the nicotinic acid contents of these foods. Nor does the wet and dry curing of meats, apart from some leaching of the vitamin which is recoverable.

PYRIDOXINE

This B vitamin (B6) is stable in the presence of heat and indeed in most cooking methods. Acids and alkalis do not affect the vitamin but significant losses can occur in all cooking methods by leaching into cooking fluids, hence these can be recovered. The losses by leaching can be 20 percent during roasting, frying and grilling; 50 percent during stewing and boiling. Fish will lose no pyridoxine during poaching; but 10 percent is leached during baking and 20 percent during frying or grilling. When vegetables are boiled, losses in all types account for 40 percent of the original content of pyridoxine but the whole of the loss can be recovered by utilizing the boiling water because all losses are due to leaching. Canned foods also will contain much of their pyridoxine in the liquid portion so this too should be used to ensure maximum intakes of the vitamin. When thawing frozen foods prior to cooking, ensure the drips are re-introduced into the diet since these too contain pyridoxine. This is relatively simple with vegetables which tend to be dropped into boiling water but may not be so obvious when meat, poultry and fish are allowed to thaw for some hours.

The only food where significant destruction of pyridoxine can occur during processing is milk. This is because at high temperatures other components of milk will react with the vitamin causing its destruction. At one time, babies fed on milk treated by high temperature processing developed pyridoxine deficiency because of this loss. When modern methods of drying milk were developed the wholesale destruction of the vitamin ceased and the problem disappeared. However, it can still occur from time to time when over zealous parents process the milk for their offspring, using excessive temperatures.

FOLIC ACID

This B vitamin occurs in foods as the free vitamin and in various combination forms. Only the free form is unstable, mainly by oxidation. Sunlight, too, can be destructive and the action of light is accelerated by riboflavin. On the other hand, vitamin C exerts a protective effect. Despite this, 30 percent of the folic acid content of tomato juice is lost when this is stored in clear glass bottles; only 7 percent of the vitamin was lost from the juice stored in dark glass bottles.

Vegetables represent a very important source of folic acid in our diets and losses can be significant during cooking processes. For example, 10 percent is lost during steam blanching; 20 percent on pressure cooking; 25 to 50 percent on boiling. Again, some of these losses are due to leaching and so can be recovered. Sterilizing milk can give rise to losses varying from 20 to 100 percent, depending on the time of contact with the air.

There are cumulative losses of folic acid in food processing. Let us consider, for example, the canning of beans. Preliminary soaking for 12 hours will leach out 5 percent after 10 minutes and 45 percent after 20 minutes, only some of which is recoverable; final sterilization in the can will destroy 10 percent of that left. This means that very little folic acid will remain in the beans once eaten by the time they are eaten.

Losses from foods such as vegetables, fruits and dairy products average 70 percent of free folic acid and 45 percent of the total of free and conjugated varieties during the overall processes of cooking. The baking of bread will destroy some 30 percent of the folic acid present in the original flour, but the final content in wholemeal bread is higher than that in white bread.

These wholesale losses of folic acid during cooking processes make it imperative, therefore, that the diet where possible should contain fresh, raw vegetables, fruits and salads to provide the requirements of this vitamin. A complete reliance on cooked and processed foods will increase the chances of a mild deficiency, particularly during pregnancy where adequate intakes of folic acid are absolutely essential for the health of the growing, unborn child.

VITAMIN B12

This is stable under most conditions but it can be destroyed by alkalis. As the vitamin is protected by the proteins of the foodstuffs and as it is confined to foods of animal origins (which are high in protein) the chances of destruction during cooking are slight. Also, the daily requirements of vitamin B12 are so small it is highly unlikely that anyone eating meat and dairy products is going to develop deficiency because of losses during cooking procedures.

PANTOTHENIC ACID

A vitamin of the B group that is stable under most cooking methods that are carried out in neutral conditions, but some destruction can occur when acids and alkalis are present. Wheat, for example, can lose as much as 60 percent of its pantothenic acid content when baking powder is used during the manufacturing process of wheat products. Meats will lose 30 percent of their pantothenic acid content when cooked but most of this is leached out and so can be recovered. Losses during the storage of deep frozen meats can be as high as 8 percent, even at these low temperatures.

BIOTIN

This B vitamin has undergone very few studies on its stability during cooking processes. It is, however, produced in very significant quantities by the bacteria that inhabit the lower end of the intestine. In view of this source therefore the behaviour of biotin and its presence in foods during the various cooking procedures is probably of little significance. However 30 percent, most of which is recoverable, is lost during the boiling of vegetables; 10 percent lost during all methods of cooking fish; 10 percent is lost when meat and poultry are cooked by any method.

The Fat Soluble Vitamins

VITAMIN A

This vitamin and its precursor carotene are insoluble in water so they do not suffer losses through extraction into processing and cooking water. The main destructive agent is oxygen but in foods both vitamins A and carotene are protected by natural antioxidants like vitamin E.

Boiling water destroys 16 percent of the vitamin A content of margarine in 30 minutes; 40 percent in one hour and 70 percent in two hours. Frying is more destructive, with losses of 40 percent in 5 minutes; 60 percent in 10 minutes and 70 percent in 15 minutes. Braising liver causes up to 10 percent loss of its vitamin A content but the level is so high to start with that this loss is not significant.

Destruction of carotene occurs when green vegetables are cooked and they can lose between 15 and 20 percent of their vitamin A activity. (Carotene functions partly by being converted to vitamin A within the body so its activity is always expressed in terms of vitamin A). Yellow vegetables lose even more with losses of between 25 and 30 percent of their vitamin A activity after freezing or canning, followed by further cooking. This is significant because it was thought until recently that canned vegetables retained all their carotene content, even after many years. These losses therefore represent a conversion of the wholly active carotene in the original vegetable to a form that is less active.

The most significant losses, totalling between 10 and 20 percent, occur when fruits and vegetables are dried under mild conditions. Even these losses are greater when traditional open-air drying is carried out and virtually complete destruction can occur.

VITAMIN D

Vitamin D is regarded as being very stable but studies are few because of the difficulty of measuring the tiny amounts of the vitamin that occur in foods. Nevertheless, the vitamin has been found to withstand the smoking of fish, the pasteurization and sterilization of milk and the drying of eggs. There are probably losses of between 25 and 35 percent of vitamin D activity during the spray-drying of milk but this is allowed for in fortification of the food with the vitamin. The significance of food contents and losses during cooking processes of vitamin D is not clear because the vitamin is also produced by the action of sunlight on the skin. However, for those who are housebound or confined indoors for other reasons, the dietary intake of vitamin D is important to their daily requirements but it does look as though eating vitamin D-rich foods, cooked or otherwise, will supply their needs.

VITAMIN E

This is very sensitive to oxidation particularly in the presence of heat and alkalis. There are serious losses in frozen foods. The most significant losses, however, are the result of the processing and refining of cereals – a very important source. Cooking foods in fats destroys between 70 and 90 percent of the vitamin E content. Greatest losses occur in the presence of rancid fats and oils and, unfortunately, these cannot always be detected by taste. Continual use of the same cooking fats and oils (e.g. in the chip pan) progressively destroys the vitamins in the food being fried. It is a sensible idea to squirt the contents of a 1000mg capsule of vitamin E into the chip pan before using the oil for chip frying. This will at least ensure that the potatoes are protected against vitamin E loss while they are being fried. Don't put the whole capsule in as the gelatine coat will not dissolve in the oil. Make sure the vitamin E you add is natural d-alpha tocopherol since this is far more efficient than the synthetic dl-variety.

Boiling vegetables like sprouts, cabbage and carrots can destroy 30 percent of their vitamin E content. When vegetables are canned even greater losses of up to 80 percent can occur. Raw vegetables and nuts are exceptionally good sources of vitamin E, so make up for the cooking losses by ensuring that these feature in your diet.

Eggs are a rather special food since, unlike other foodstuffs mentioned above, eggs when cooked are unlikely to lose any vitamins by leaching. The rapid coagulation of the egg albumen protein during the cooking process tends to retain them all and, of course, when boiled the shell acts as a barrier. Losses are therefore all due to destruction of the vitamins and these can vary from 30 percent in fried eggs down to 10 percent in boiled of folic acid; 20 percent in fried down to 10 percent in boiled of thiamine;

20 percent in poached, scrambled or omelette down to 5 percent in boiled of riboflavine; 20 percent in fried down to 10% in boiled of pyridoxine and 20 percent in fried down to 10 percent in boiled of pantothenic acid. Amounts destroyed by poaching, scrambling or omelette are similar for all vitamins.

3 | Looking to your diet

The food we eat remains the prime source of the vitamins we need and a careful selection of dietary items will ensure at least the minimum requirements of those essential micronutrients. This applies only under normal conditions of living however and as we shall see, lifestyles, habits, medicinal drugs, cooking methods, storage of food, digestive ability and many other factors can cause losses of vitamins or an increased body requirement. Self-help must therefore come first by considering the type of food we eat and the way we treat it before it is eaten. All natural food contains some vitamins and by eating a balanced mixture of food items a wide spectrum of vitamin intake will be obtained. Let us look, therefore, at the general principles of food levels of vitamins.

Dietary sources of vitamins

CEREALS

These comprise an important part of the diet for their energy contribution to the body and for their dietary fibre content. They include grains, flours, starches, breakfast cereals, biscuits, cakes, buns, pastries and puddings. As cereal products tend to be eaten in large quantities their contribution of protein is also not insignificant. They supply excellent quantities of the vitamin B complex, apart from vitamin B12, but are completely devoid of vitamins A, D, C and the provitamin beta-carotene. Hence we must look to other food items to supply these missing vitamins

Despite the usefulness of cereals and cereal products as suppliers of the B vitamins (apart from B12) and indeed of vitamin E, the levels are reduced quite drastically by the refining and processing of the foods as provided by nature into the type that most of us eat. Whole grains and wholemeal flour represent the best unrefined cereals that we have in our diet, in the form of mueslis and wholemeal bread, which still retain their full complement of B vitamins (apart from vitamin B12) and vitamin E. Of course, when a wheatgrain is refined, the material removed such as the bran and wheatgerm, is usually richer in all the vitamins present than the original grain because the vitamins tend to be concentrated in those parts removed. Although we like to think of wheatbran as an excellent source of dietary fibre we should remember that it is also a rich provider of most of the B vitamins and vitamin E. Wheatgerm also is a highly significant source of these vitamins particularly in respect of vitamins B1 and E. Taken in isolation, all types of bran and cereal germs are very rich in the B vitamins (but not B12) and in vitamin E. For this reason they should be regarded, and indeed are by many people, as food supplements that can be added to other foods to enhance their vitamin levels.

Cooked items of cereal-based foods such as bread, cakes, biscuits, buns, pastries and puddings will also provide useful intakes of the vitamins present in the original cereals but will of necessity be at lower levels because of the cooking processes used. The addition of water and sugar, which do not provide vitamins to cooked cereal products will also dilute somewhat the vitamin content of the original cereals. White sugar supplies 'empty' calories, which means energy without the accompanying vitamins and minerals; brown and raw sugar do however contain some vitamins, as indeed does honey, but their contribution is not significant.

MILK AND MILK PRODUCTS

Milk has been described as the complete food since it contains all the main dietary constituents carbohydrate, fat and protein, plus a full spectrum of all the necessary vitamins and minerals needed for health. All it lacks is dietary fibre. This applies to whole milk but this can be subdivided into a fatty and an aqueous phase. Not surprisingly, therefore, the fatty or creamy part is rich in the fat soluble vitamins A, D and E and in the provitamin beta-carotene. Skimmed milk which comprises the main aqueous part of liquid milk, is therefore much richer in the water-soluble B vitamins complex and vitamin C and is virtually devoid of the fat-soluble vitamins. As butter is a concentrated form of milk fat it is an excellent source of all the fat-soluble vitamins (although, of course, butter, cream and full-cream milk are high in animal fats which raise the level of cholesterol in the blood); by a similar token dried skimmed milk supplies excellent quantities of all the B vitamins and vitamin C because they are concentrated by the removal of water. Similarly, cheese and yoghurt, produced from milk, retain the vitamin contents of the starting material. Indeed, since both are fermentation products it is possible for them, particularly yoghurt, to contain more B vitamins because of synthesis during the fermentative process. Milk, cheese and yoghurt are the sole significant sources of vitamin B12 in the diet of lactovegetarians who should ensure that these foods feature as part of their diet.

The practice of adding milk or cream to our cereals and mueslis therefore has some logic in providing a combination food that supplies a useful balance of all the vitamins needed in the diet. With the present-day trend of replacing whole milk by the skimmed variety to cut down dairy fat intake, to prevent the build-up of a high level of cholesterol related to heart disease, a valuable source of fat-soluble vitamins has been lost. It is essential, therefore, to make up this deficit by seeking out other foods to supply these essential fatty micronutrients.

FATS AND OILS

These food constituents can be disregarded as sources of all the B vitamins and vitamin C. They are, however, significant providers of the fat-soluble vitamins. In fact vegetable oils represent our most important dietary source of vitamin E. Not all vegetable oils contain the vitamin, for example, olive and coconut oils are virtually free of it, and this probably reflects the fact that these oils do not contain very much polyunsaturated fatty acids. It is a fact of nature that in general the higher the content of these essential fatty acids in an oil, the higher is the vitamin E content. The vitamin functions in the seed or nut that contain these oils as a protecting agent of the polyunsaturated fatty acids. Similarly, cod liver oil, which is a rich source of these acids, is also high in vitamin E content.

In the absence of vitamin E, these polyunsaturated oils soon become rancid. Unfortunately, the processing required to extract these dietary oils like maize (corn), sunflower, safflower and soya, from the appropriate seed or grain will destroy or remove the vitamin E. Once the protective vitamin is removed and if it is not replaced, the oils break down rapidly when used in cooking processes and the resulting products can be quite toxic. Ensure, therefore, that the vegetable oil you buy contains vitamin E – if the vitamin is mentioned on the label you may assume it has been added and is perfectly acceptable.

Fats that have been produced from animal or fish sources contain vitamins A, D and E, although compound cooking fat and lard are virtually free of them because they have been processed out. The richest source of vitamins A and D are the fish liver oils but they can hardly be regarded as frequent or regular constituents of the diet. These oils can instead be taken in capsule form or by the teaspoonful as supplementary vitamins A and D.

Vitamin A as such does not actually occur in plant foods. However, vegetarians and vegans (extreme vegetarians) can obtain adequate intakes by means of the carotene which is in plants as the body is able to convert this into the vitamin as needed. Similarly, vitamin D does not occur in the commonly eaten plant foods. Despite the wide occurrence of carotene in plant foods, vegetable oils used in cooking or eaten raw on salads, contain only traces. The exception is unrefined palm oil, which is an extremely rich source of carotene, but this oil is hardly a common item of diet. The lack of vitamins A, D and carotene in edible vegetable oils means that when these are hardened and hence converted into margarine the resulting fat is devoid of these vitamins. For this reason, legislation now demands that all margarines are fortified with vitamin A or carotene and vitamin D to bring their levels up to those of butter. Vitamin E is readily destroyed by the hardening process that converts vegetable oils to margarines and often this vitamin too is added to these fats, although present legislation does not demand it. You should look for vitamin E, printed on the label and ensure that your brand contains it.

MEAT AND MEAT PRODUCTS

Muscle meats and products made from them are poor providers of vitamins A, D and carotene. They all contain some vitamin E but the concentrations are way below those found in vegetable oils. Most offal too is a poor source of vitamin A and carotene, but the vitamin E levels are somewhat higher than those in muscle meats. The exceptions are liver and kidney which provide very large amounts of vitamin A combined with significant intakes of vitamin D. Vitamin B levels are no higher than offal. Carotene contents vary amongst the livers from species and usually reflect the diet of the animal.

All muscle meats contain the whole spectrum of the water–soluble vitamin B complex but there is no vitamin C present at all. Again we must look to offal, particularly the liver and kidney, for the really rich providers of the vitamins – this time the B complex. Unlike muscle meats, all offal supplies useful quantities of vitamin C in the raw state but these tend to be reduced somewhat during cooking processes.

One of the most important B vitamins that we get from meat products is vitamin B12. These foodstuffs represent our most significant source of the vitamin and if these are not eaten as part of the diet, the chances of deficiency are increased. Lactovegetarians at least obtain their needs from dairy products (including eggs) but vegans should look to supplementation with the vitamin to ensure they are not deficient. Fortunately, unlike most B vitamins, substantial quantities of vitamin B12 are stored within the liver. The daily needs are so low (in the nature of one millionth of one gram) that once liver levels are built up, there is ample present for some time. The best way to accumulate vitamin B12 rapidly is to have it injected directly into the muscle but as this is the medical rather than the dietary approach, it is beyond the scope of readers of this book. Nevertheless, many vegans choose this method of taking their vitamin B12 in preference to a daily oral intake because injections are infrequent. Nevertheless, injection of the vitamin is the only solution if you are unable to absorb the vitamin from the diet. This condition, however, requires professional diagnosis and treatment.

POULTRY AND GAME

Apart from vitamin C which is not present in any poultry and game foods, all the vitamins are provided in significant quantities by these foodstuffs. The concentrations are similar to those of meats derived from animals.

FISH AND SEAFOODS

As eaten, white fish like cod, haddock, sole, plaice, halibut and whiting provide trace quantities only of vitamins A, D and of carotene. Some vitamin E is present but levels are rarely above one milligram per 100g (3.5oz). The only significant vitamins provided are those of the B complex and particularly vitamin B12. The quantity of vitamin C present in all these species is negligible. White fish should therefore be regarded primarily as good providers of the B vitamins only.

Fatty fish are different. Hence eels, herrings, bloaters, kippers, mackerel, pilchards, salmon, sardines, sprats, trout, tuna and whitebait are all useful suppliers of vitamins A, D and E but contain only traces of carotene. All the B vitamins are provided by these fish, at levels comparable to those in white wish, apart from vitamin B12 which occurs at much higher concentrations in fatty fish. Hence, apart from vitamin C, which is present in negligible quantities, the fatty fish provide the whole spectrum of vitamins in significant amounts. In this respect they are superior to white fish.

Cartilaginous fish, like dogfish and skate, provide few vitamins apart from members of the B complex and vitamin E.

Despite the fact that they are often regarded as delicacies, crustacea such as crab, lobster, prawns and shrimps provide little in the way of vitamins. Their main attributes are the presence of the vitamin B complex and of vitamin E, but levels are low relative to those fish and of meats. Molluscs like cockles, mussels, scallops and whelks too are not very rich providers of the vitamin B complex but do contain useful quantities of vitamin E. The only exception is oysters which supply significant quantities of vitamin A and higher levels of the vitamin B complex than do other molluscs.

VEGETABLES

All vegetables provide the whole range of B vitamins apart from B12 and. although the concentrations are low, the relatively large amounts of vegetables eaten in the normal diet mean that they are an important source of these vitamins. Some high concentrations are however found in butter beans, haricot beans, mung beans, lentils, peas and potatoes, all of which are relatively rich in thiamine, riboflavin, nicotinic acid and pyridoxine, and the green-leafed vegetables are important providers of folic acid. Vegetarians are less likely than meat-eaters to be deficient in this B vitamin because of their high intake of leaf vegetables.

No vegetables contain vitamin A but all will provide carotene, the orange colouring agent which the body is able to convert into vitamin A. Even green vegetables contain carotene but its colour is masked by the stronger — coloured green chlorophyll. Hence green beans, brussels sprouts, broccoli, cabbage, lettuce, peas, spinach, spring greens, turnip tops, asparagus and watercress all are rich sources of carotene. When chlorophyll is absent, as in carrots, corn, sweet potatoes and tomatoes, the natural orange or yellow colour of carotene becomes more obvious and all are excellent providers of the vitamin A precursor. Vitamin D is however absent in vegetables. Most contain some vitamin E and, in view of the large amounts of vegetables eaten in the usual diet, significant quantities of the vitamin are obtained from these foodstuffs.

There is considerable variation in vitamin C contents amongst the vegetables but, as a general rule, the green-leafed varieties are richer than the beans, peas and root vegetables. The contribution of all vegetables in a good, mixed diet to our vitamin C intake is however significant. Potatoes are not a particularly rich source, especially when they are old, but in the Western world where they represent a staple part of the diet the sheer bulk eaten provides our main source of the vitamin. As most slimming regimes tend to avoid potatoes it is important to ensure other sources of vitamin C like vegetables and fruits are eaten to compensate for its lack in those undergoing such diets. New potatoes as picked are good providers of vitamin C but 80 percent can be lost as they age. Raw green peppers represent the richest vegetable source of vitamin C.

FRUITS

Like vegetables, fruits do not contain any vitamin A, but this is compensated by wide-ranging contents of the vitamin precursor carotene. Similarly fruits, like vegetables, do not contain any vitamin B12 or vitamin D, but there are unconfirmed reports that the latter vitamin is present in avocado pears. The rest of the B complex vitamins are present in all fruits, albeit at fairly low concentrations. Fruits also supply small amounts of vitamin E which, whilst useful as part of a varied diet, do not represent a particularly significant source when taken alone.

Although we tend to regard fruits as excellent sources of vitamin C, its concentration varies over a wide range in the various species. Pride of place goes to blackcurrants, gooseberries, oranges, grapefruit, lemons and limes, with pineapples also good providers of the vitamin. Unfortunately, the vitamin does not survive the drying process in the production of dried fruits which are virtually devoid of it. Apples provide varying quantities depending upon the variety – Sturmer Pippin represents the richest source, with Cox's at the other end of the scale.

NUTS

All nuts may be regarded as good sources of the B vitamins, with the exception of vitamin B12. They also feature as the richest sources of vitamin E amongst all foodstuffs. They are however completely lacking in vitamins A, D and carotene, and vitamin C levels are so low as to be disregarded. Roasted nuts however do tend to have lower levels of the B vitamins because of losses induced during the roasting process.

OTHER FOODS

Sugar, confectionery, jams, fruit spreads, marmalades, honey and preserves all provide only negligible quantities of the B vitamins and carotene or none at all. Jams and preserves contain some vitamin C provided by the fruit content but concentrations are not high. Chocolate products do provide reasonable amounts of the B vitamins, and vitamin E mainly by virtue of their cocoa and vegetable fat contents.

Beverages contain traces only of the B vitamins (apart from vitamin B12) with the exception of coffee which is a rich source of nicotinic acid. Instant coffee can contain as much as 39mg of this vitamin per 100g (3.5oz). Similarly, fruit juices provide only trace amounts of the B vitamins but their content of vitamin C is high enough to represent an important source of this vitamin.

Beers, lagers and wines all provide a wide spectrum of the B vitamins produced mainly during the fermentation process. Spirits, however, are completely devoid of all vitamins.

Soups will add some vitamins to the daily diet but the amounts present depend very much on the ingredients. Vegetables, meats and fowl that provide vitamins in their original state will also contribute them to the soup but the amount of processing the soup has been through will determine how many survive. When prepared from dried powders, the resulting soup is usually less nutritious in terms of its vitamin content than one of the tinned variety or, better still, one made from fresh ingredients.

Yeast is regarded as a good source of the B vitamins (apart from vitamin B12) particularly when it is dried. However, although a useful supplement, when taken in tablet form or sprinkled on food, dried yeast should not be regarded as a sole source of B vitamins since 100g (3.5oz) would have to be eaten daily to provide requirements. Most people could not tolerate the strong taste of this amount and at this level yeast could induce gout in susceptible people. Yeast should therefore be regarded simply as a useful vitamin B supplement when taken at the recommended dose.

Similarly, yeast extracts, which are concentrated from dried yeast, are extremely rich sources of the B vitamins (apart from vitamin B12, unless this is added) but they tend to be eaten in small amounts. Nevertheless, even at this level, they are very useful vitamin B supplements. Beef extracts will also provide excellent intakes of the B vitamins with the added advantage that they contain much more vitamin B12 than yeast extracts.

Non-dietary source of vitamins

Usually we tend to regard the diet as the main source of our vitamin needs under normal circumstances but some of them are supplied from non-dietary sources. Nicotinic acid, for example, can be made within body cells, particularly the liver, from the essential amino acid l-tryptophane. Although we define a vitamin as being an essential micronutrient that can be supplied only in the food, nicotinic acid is the exception. It is extremely doubtful that our complete requirements of nicotinic acid could be met by body synthesis from l-tryptophane because the rate of conversion is very inefficient. It has been calculated that it requires 60mg l-tryptophane to produce just 1 mg of nicotinic acid. Nevertheless this source can become significant when the vitamin is not being supplied directly in sufficient quantity by the diet. It must be said however that a diet poor in nicotinic acid is also likely to be poor also in good quality protein which supplies our dietary needs of l-tryptophane. Remember too that this amino acid has many other functions within the body, not only as a building block of tissue protein but as a precursor of brain substances needed for normal brain and nerve function. Its function as a precursor that can be converted to nicotinic acid must be regarded as minor but one that can assume importance when other sources of the vitamin are lacking. Good quality protein (e.g. from eggs, milk, meats, poultry, pulses, grains and seeds) will supply plenty of l-tryptophane enough to provide a useful supplementary supply of the vitamin.

Vitamin D is also synthesised within the body tissues by the action of sunlight upon the skin. Indeed this can supply such a proportion of the body's needs that it has been suggested that vitamin D should not be regarded as a vitamin at all! Whilst this may be true in those fortunate enough to live in a sunny climate all years round, many of those of us who do not will still require dietary sources of the vitamin. In fact one of the reasons why the vitamin D deficiency disease rickets appear in epidemic proportions in the industrial area of the UK and the rest of Europe was that the polluted air prevented the sunlight from falling on the skin of those living in these areas. When this factor was coupled with a poor intake of foods rich in the vitamin, perhaps it is not surprising deficiency developed.

The moral here is obvious. If you live in a cool climate ensure that whenever possible you get out into the sunshine so your body can make its own vitamin D. This vitamin is fat-soluble which means that it can be stored within the liver and fatty tissues of the body. The importance of this storage of vitamin D from the vitamin produced by the action of sunlight on the skin was demonstrated recently in a study of children from the East End of London. Half the children from one particular school were given two weeks' holiday at the seaside during the summer months. The other half stayed at home. All the children received a similar diet with virtually identical intakes of vitamin D from their food throughout the year. Six months after their summer holiday, those children who had spent just two weeks at the seaside had significantly higher levels of blood vitamin D than those who had stayed at home. A good insurance policy, then, is to build up your vitamin D supplies during the sunny weather by exposing the skin to the sun to stand you in good stead in the winter months when sunshine is less apparent. (Too much sunbathing is, of course, bad for the skin and can cause sunburn and even skin cancer). Look also to your dietary intakes during the winter, making sure your diet contains vitamin D-rich foods and even supplementing your diet with fish-liver-oils.

At the lower end of the large intestine there is a thriving population of bacteria which helps in the digestive and elimination processes. In fact about half of normal faeces consists of these bacteria which are eliminated along with waste good products. The bacteria, which are harmless, are usually nicely balanced to prevent over-production of the harmful bacteria and of the yeasts which can cause disease if allowed to flourish. Thrush is a good example of an infection due to yeasts which have been allowed to overproduce when the controlling effect of the 'friendly bacteria' has been lost. Lactobacilli represent one of the more important 'friendly bacteria' and as these are supplied in ample quantity by a living yoghurt the advantages of this food are obvious.

The introduction of powerful antibiotics to treat infective disease has however been shown to affect adversely the population of friendly bacteria that live in the large intestine. In addition to the pathogenic (harmful) bacteria that are destroyed by these antibiotics, the intestinal bacteria are also killed off, with the result that some vitamins normally synthesized by them are no longer available to the body. This is because such bacteria have the ability to make vitamins for their own use which can later be absorbed and utilized by the body. Amongst the vitamins known to be produced by the intestinal bacteria are biotin, pantothenic acid and vitamin K. We know this because studies have indicated that people can excrete more of these vitamins than was present in the food eaten. The excess must therefore have been supplied within the intestinal tract. Also it is known that long-term antibiotic treatment can give rise to deficiencies of biotin and of vitamin K because these vitamins are no longer being supplied by the intestinal bacteria. When dietary intakes of these vitamins are low, their synthesis by the 'friendly bacteria' then assumes great importance. It is likely that all the vitamins are made to some extent by the 'friendly bacteria' but most of them, with the exception of those mentioned above, are either produced in such low potency as to be of little help to the host or they are produced too far down the intestinal tract to be absorbed.

Recent studies though have indicated that in some people, the intestinal bacteria can provide significant quantities of vitamin B12 that can be absorbed and made available to the host. Usually the vitamin cannot be assimilated because when produced in this way it is too far down the intestine to be absorbed. Some people, however, for one reason or another have bacterial populations that live much higher up in the intestinal tract than is usual – so high in fact that the vitamin B12 produced can be utilized. Such people are those who live in areas of the world where the standard of hygiene is lower perhaps than that desired by more fortunate populations, in other words the inhabitants of most Third World countries. This goes a long way in explaining why such individuals, whilst lacking the B12-rich foods like meats and dairy products in their diets nevertheless do not develop vitamin B12 deficiency. Similarly, it now looks as if vegans and other extreme vegetarians may, because of their diet, develop bacterial populations higher up the intestine than meat-eaters and so benefit from locally-produced vitamin B12. However, vegans in particular would be well advised to take a supplementary form of vitamin B12 daily. This is because bacterial synthesis may produce just enough of the vitamin to prevent the symptoms of deficiency but it may not suffice to provide the quantity required for optimum health.

The best example of complete synthesis of vitamin needs within the body is provided by ruminants like cattle, sheep and goats. These animals possess a rumen, one of their four stomachs, that acts like a fermentation tank. Within this, the bacterial population produces all the members of the vitamin B complex from nutrients supplied in the forage. Although some of these vitamins are introduced in the diet, significant quantities are produced within the rumen. Vitamin B12 is synthesized in large quantity by this natural process so these animals are highly unlikely to suffer a deficiency even though the vitamin is not supplied in their vegetarian diet. The only time that ruminants may be prone to vitamin B12 deficiency is when the soil on which they graze, and hence the food that they eat, is deficient in the mineral cobalt. When this is lacking, the rumen bacteria cannot synthesize vitamin B12.

4 | Nutritional causes of deficiency

Poor storage of food, cooking methods that do not retain the full vitamin potency of food items and inefficient utilization of cooking fluids can all cause significant losses of vitamins. In addition there are many other factors that can give rise to vitamin deficiency and most individuals will be prone to the influence of one or more. Let us now consider these so that if you can identify them as being relevant to yourself you will be able to take steps to remedy any potential deficiency.

APATHY

This is often a feature of people living alone, within all age groups, but particularly in those who have lost a spouse and perhaps no longer have a family to look after. There is little incentive to prepare adequate meals which are often monotonous and not nourishing enough. Impaired digestive ability may be associated with the apathy and this may exacerbate the low nutritional status of the individual. The apathetic approach to eating is often seen in the elderly middle-aged bachelor or spinster living in accommodation with poor cooking facilities, or in teenagers and students who are living alone for the first time. The obvious remedy is to pay more attention to the diet in conjunction perhaps with an all-round multivitamin supplement.

DENTAL PROBLEMS

Poor dentition, for whatever reason, whether loss of teeth, dental decay or ill-fitting dentures, can make eating uncomfortable. The result is an aversion to foods that require a lot of chewing, such as salads, meats and vegetables. As these food items are important suppliers of the whole range of vitamins needed, the chances of deficiency developing are increased when they are not provided in the diet. A filling, though ill-balanced diet, must inevitably lead to a mild deficiency of vitamins. Poor dental health will contribute to it, so improving this must be the first step in ensuring a well-balanced and hence healthier diet.

FOOD FADS

Nutritional imbalances are often seen when excessive quantities of particular items of food, usually of the 'empty-calorie' variety, are eaten at the expense of other more nutritionally desirable foodstuffs. Young people are particularly prone to this factor of imbalance when they prefer high calorie but low vitamin content foods, such as sugar-rich foods, soft drinks, confectionery, potato snacks, sweets, cakes and the like, to more basic but less attractive (at least to them) foods. Old people are not immune to food fad diets either and will often partake of excessive intakes of beverages, processed cereals and preserves to the detriment of more nourishing foods. The food fads sometimes associated with pregnancy do not have the same significance because they are variable and usually of a temporary nature. It has been suggested that they may be satisfying a demand by the woman for specific nutrients and so should not be discouraged. Other food fads should, however, be regarded as contributing to an insidious development of mild vitamin deficiencies and should be treated by improving the diet or, failing this, by at least ensuring the minimum daily requirements of these micronutrients with a good multivitamin preparations.

FOOD TABOOS

They tend to arise because of religious beliefs but these, in turn, are often a logical response to knowledge about the food based on bitter experience. Meat that is prone to parasitic infection is often avoided for obvious reason but there can be unwanted results. For example, when pork is taboo, the richest meat source of thiamine is denied and the chances of developing a mild deficiency are increased accordingly. Dairy products based on cow's milk are often avoided avidly by some people but in so doing they are depriving themselves of a rich source of vitamin D and the B complex vitamin B2. Unless other food sources of these are eaten, a mild deficiency will develop. Some people, of course, are genuinely afraid of products based on cow's milk because of allergic reactions to them so they must look to other ways of obtaining these vitamins.

Those who do not eat meat or poultry products (or even fish) like vegetarians and those who are even more extreme like those who avoid all food products of animal origin may also be regarded as food faddists. Their main concern should be their intake of dietary vitamin B12 which is available to really significant amounts only from foods of animal origin. They should be aware that vitamin B12 deficiency, and, in the case of vegans, riboflavin deficiency is far more likely because of their dietary habits. The supplementary vitamin, made by fermentation and hence of non-animal source, is essential for them to receive optimal intakes.

In some cases of food taboos, specific foods that are nutritionally sound are avoided because of an unfounded belief that they do harm. Many such beliefs abound in Africa, South America and the Far East. In Bolivia, for example, any food containing animal blood is believed to make children mute so it is avoided during pregnancy by the mother and withheld from the child after birth. In West Pakistan, buffalo milk is quite erroneously believed to produce great physical strength but to reduce the mental ability of the person who drinks it. Hence a nutritious food is avoided by many — a situation made even more tragic when this food represents a potentially important source of protein, vitamins and minerals. Unfortunately, in these parts of the world many food taboos are confined to the pregnant woman who is thus often deprived of the very nutrients she desperately requires.

FASTING

Complete avoidance of food or fasting is often a feature of many religious sects. The occasional 24-hour fast, believed by some to be a useful practice in purging the body of toxins and poisons, probably does little harm in terms of reducing vitamin intakes. Where extensive fasting is undertaken as in Ramadan, however, there is almost certainly nutritional harm done. Whether this affects the health and eventual life span of Moslem people has not been studied, but logic would suggest that the lack of vitamins and minerals taken in over long periods must deplete their levels in the body. Water-soluble vitamins, because they are not stored to any great extent, are the most likely to be depleted during prolonged fasting. Fat soluble vitamins are stored in the liver and fatty tissues of the body so during periods of normal eating, sufficient of these are retained to supply requirements when food intake is stopped.

INDIVIDUAL REQUIREMENTS

These are usually expressed by official bodies as recommended dietary intakes or as recommended daily allowances. They are regarded as sufficient to prevent symptoms of deficiency diseases but not necessarily sufficient to maintain optimum health. Three criteria are used to assess these levels:

1. They take account of individual variations in requirements by introducing a safety factor to cover 95 per cent of the population.
2. They take account of possible increase caused by the minor stresses of life but extra needs during infection, injuries and other illnesses are ignored.
3. They are unlikely to take account of different availability of vitamins in various foods.

Despite these assurances, the wide range of suggested daily intakes amongst various countries with similar ethnic groups would suggest that none of them are really aware of what our needs are. Why, for example, do the Russians and Rumanians regard 75 to 85mg vitamin C as a desirable daily intake, while in the United Kingdom only 30mg is regarded as adequate? Similarly, these Eastern Bloc countries suggest that vitamin A needs for their people are twice those that the Department of Health in the UK regarded as sufficient for Britons. Fortunately, the EC recommendations coming into force are more realistic intakes.

Experiments indicate that animals of the same species can vary one from another in their vitamin requirements by anything from two to ten-fold. Often, although the lower figures represents what is needed to prevent abject signs of deficiency, the higher figure is that required for optimum health. A similar situation applies also to human beings. Two people on a similar diet can show wide variation in their blood levels of vitamins, suggesting that individual human needs are also different. Hence the individual with the higher requirements can be suffering from a mild deficiency of some vitamins simply because his requirements are not met from a diet that would supply adequate intakes for someone else. Without extensive testing no one can determine their exact requirements with any accuracy but if benefit is felt from an all-round vitamin supplement taken regularly, it would suggest that their needs are not met by the diet.

To illustrate varying official views on what their people need in the way of daily vitamin intakes, the following figures are taken from American, UK, USSR and EC authorities respectively:

OFFICIAL RECOMMENDED DAILY VITAMIN INTAKES

	USA	UK	USSR	EC
VITAMIN A (µg)	750	1,000	1,500	800
VITAMIN D (µg)	7.0	2.5	10	5.0
VITAMIN E (mg)	15	–	–	10
THIAMIN (mg)	1.4	1.1	1.8	1.4
RIBOFLAVIN (mg)	1.6	1.7	2.4	1.6
NICOTINIC ACID (mg)	20	19	25	18
PANTOTHENIC ACID(mg)	7.0	–	10.0	6.0
PYRIDOXINE (mg)	2.0	–	2.1	2.0
BIOTIN (mg)	100	–	–	150
FOLIC ACID (µg)	400	300	500	200
VITAMIN B12 (µg)	3.5	2.0	5.0	1.0
VITAMIN C (mg)	45	30	80	60

N.B. Blanks indicate that no particular level is recommended.

These figures should be regarded merely as a guideline. There is no reason why with a good diet they not be doubled at least. The higher the intake the more likely it is that requirements for optimum health are achieved, at least up to certain limits. When the diet cannot supply such needs, supplementation then becomes essential.

OTHER FOOD NUTRIENTS

The need for vitamins may be increased by other food constituents. Vitamin levels may also be reduced under the influence of other nutrients. Prime examples of these factors are seen with high polyunsaturated fats intakes, a trend that is increasing amongst the health-conscious public. Unless the requisite vitamin E is taken at the same time, high levels of these fats can induce deficiency of the vitamin. In fact, the simplest way to make experimental animals vitamin E deficient in order to study the effects, is to feed large amounts of polyunsaturated vegetable oils that are devoid of the vitamin. Not only is their vitamin E intake decreased but the body levels of the vitamin are drastically reduced.

Any increase in dietary calories, especially of the empty kind, will need a concomitant rise in thiamine intake as the two are related. When the vitamin in the diet does not keep pace with these empty calories, a mild deficiency will gradually develop. This is probably one of the main causes of the widespread increase in mild thiamine deficiency that is being observed today in the Western world.

In a similar manner, high dietary intakes of protein should be accompanied by increased vitamin B6 in the diet. Fortunately, high protein foods tend to contain high B6 levels, but if these are destroyed by poor cooking techniques or other destructive factors, an imbalance will occur. Alternatively, when protein intakes are low, less vitamin B6 is required.

Specific amino acids in the diet (as part of the food protein) can also influence vitamin levels. We have seen that low tryptophane levels in the diet can reduce nicotinic acid concentrations because the amino acids act as a precursor of the vitamin. At the same time, another amino acid, leucine, when present in high-dietary concentrations needs extra nicotinic acid. A food high in leucine and low in tryptophane, such as millet, is therefore conducive to nicotinic acid deficiency. Hence, in those countries where millet is the staple diet, the chances of this particular deficiency are increased.

Some proteins can cause inactivation or destruction of vitamins. Avidin is a protein unique to raw egg-white that combines with and inactivates the B-vitamin biotin. When the egg-white is cooked, avidin is destroyed so the full potency of the vitamin is available. The moral is to avoid high intakes of raw egg-white.

Another food that can cause destruction of vitamins is raw fish. The reason is that this foodstuff contains an enzyme called thiaminase which specifically destroys thiamine. Thiaminase, like all enzymes, is protein in nature so it is destroyed when the food containing it is cooked. In some parts of the world, notably the Far East, raw fish is a staple part of the diet so the chances of this inducing a thiamine deficiency are increased. At the same time thiamine can be easily inactivated by a bacterium called Bacillus thiaminolyticus which is a common infective micro-organism of raw fish. A combination of these two factors in the diet of Japanese is believed to be the reason why three percent of the population suffer mild deficiency of thiamine. In the West where we tend to cook our fish before eating it, the problems do not arise because both the thiaminase and the microorganism are destroyed by the cooking process.

OTHER VITAMINS

Excessive intakes of one vitamin may induce deficiency of another. Such situations may not arise very often in everyday life but it has been established that very high intakes of folic acid can cause a deficiency of vitamin B12. This can happen in vegetarians and in particular vegans, who combine high dietary levels of folic acid (present in vegetables) with much reduced intakes of vitamin B12 (present in fish, animal foods and dairy products). An imbalance of folic acid and vitamin B12 intakes in the daily diet can also lead to clinical complications. If a vegetarian or vegan loses the ability to absorb vitamin B12, their high folic acid intake will mask the anaemia caused by deficiency of the B12. What is not masked is the insidious degeneration of the spinal cord that is an additional feature of vitamin B12 deficiency. A stage is eventually reached when the nervous system is damaged beyond repair. It is therefore important that vitamin B12 deficiency is diagnosed rapidly in vegans and vegetarians and this is the province of the medical practitioner. For this reason, too, the availability of the vitamin B12 and folic acid in products on sale to the public is confined to those containing only a low potency. This is to avoid overdosage with folic acid masking a possible deficiency of vitamin B12.

Other vitamin interactions that have been observed are high levels of carotene inducing a vitamin D deficiency when vitamin D intakes are on the borderline. When vitamin C is missing, folic acid deficiency symptoms can manifest themselves. This is because vitamin C is essential for the folic acid in the body to be converted to its metabolic active form, folinic acid. Even if folic acid is present at high concentration it is useless unless there is sufficient vitamin C available to activate it. Both vitamins must therefore be present for folic acid-deficiency anaemia to be avoided.

5 | Population sectors that are likely to be vitamin deficient

A vitamin deficiency can occur in two ways. In the first, a primary deficiency can be caused by an inadequate diet resulting in a reduced intake over a long period of time. This may be months or years in the case of those vitamins like A and B12 which are stored to a great extent during periods of adequate intakes. Most vitamins, however, have a high turnover which means that a deficiency manifests itself fairly quickly once intakes start to drop.

In the second way a conditioned deficiency arises out of an adequate diet where other factors affect the vitamin intake. These factors may decrease the absorption of vitamins; prevent their release from the food eaten; cause increased requirements over and above those in an adequate diet; increase their turnover; or give rise to enhanced excretion. In the previous section these factors were discussed but it is because they can induce deficiency that many authorities are now questioning the concept of an average vitamin intake from the diet. It is quite likely that each individual has his or her vitamin requirements peculiar to themselves. These can, of course, fall below those recommended as the norm but it is more likely they will be higher.

Hence it is now recognised that not only individuals can vary in their vitamin requirements but there do exist various sectors in the population who by their very nature are likely to need more vitamins to maintain health. Although these extra vitamin needs could, in theory, be met by improving the diet, in many cases this is not always possible or practicable, so supplementary sources must be sought. In addition, some people's need for vitamins is so high that there is no way these levels can be obtained even from a very good diet.

Many nutritional studies have indicated which sectors of the population are likely to require vitamins and these will now be discussed. If you find you fit into one of these population sectors, the chances are that you should be looking to your vitamin intake. The benefits obtained by a diet change or simple supplementation will outweigh any nominal cost involved.

Are you elderly?

Various studies on vitamins in the elderly have drawn attention to many aspects of nutrition in those of advancing years. No one is quite sure of their vitamin requirements, nor do they know to what extent these vitamins are absorbed from the food eaten. It is highly likely that the efficiency of absorption decreases as a person ages, so naturally more must be eaten. This was demonstrated quite clearly in one study where old people living in an institution were eating an adequate diet with ample vitamin levels yet their body content was invariably low. Only by a general vitamin supplementation were body levels of vitamins restored to where they should have been. One note of interest was the immediate benefit to health experienced.

Other factors contributing to a decreased intake of micronutrients in old people include a host of social, psychological and economic influences. Some more specific problems in this area are poor dentition leading to an aversion to vitamin-rich foods like salads, whole grains and meat; a reluctance for physical or emotional reasons to shop frequently for a wide variety of foodstuffs; loss of a spouse leading to a reluctance to cook food, with undue reliance on refined carbohydrates and beverages of doubtful nutritional value; excessive losses of vitamin due to the methods used in mass cooking of meals where these form the staple diet. All these factors can reduce vitamin intake.

Vitamin malnutrition may lead to a much worse state of affairs resulting in a phase of sub-clinical nutrition which can lead to poor health, apathy and disinterest – a vicious circle too common in elderly people. The most common deficiencies encountered were those of vitamin B1 (thiamine), vitamin C and vitamins A and D. The problem has reached such a level that the writer of a leading article in the *British Medical Journal* feels it would be beneficial to offer people of an advanced age supplements like liquid milk fortified with vitamin D. This would be a useful source of vitamins and minerals as well as the milk protein and calories which older people may also lack.

It would also be beneficial to any old person to be given iron, vitamin B complex, vitamin C and the fat-soluble vitamins A and D for some weeks following an illness or operation. Vitamins are needed for overcoming the effects of illness and for the rapid healing of wounded tissue and any lack of these nutrients to the aged must have a deleterious effect upon recovery.

A report of the Panel on Nutrition of the Elderly drew attention to the fact that the lack of sunlight falling onto the skin of housebound old people would predispose them to a deficiency of vitamin D, leading to softening of the bones, a disease called osteomalacia. This condition, the adult counterpart of childhood rickets, may also be complicated by osteoporosis — a literal honeycombing of the bone leading to easy breakage. It now looks like an adequate intake of vitamin D and calcium throughout life will reduce considerably the chances of developing these conditions in old age. Vitamin D is best taken to prevent the development of osteomalacia and osteoporosis, which you can do on a self-help basis rather than wait for the diseases to appear and then be treated professionally.

Many studies indicate that vitamin C intakes in the elderly are low and these are reflected in the findings that body levels in these people are also reduced. Although few overt signs of scurvy appear, these low levels probably contribute to the generalised malaise often observed in the elderly — a condition that usually responds to simple supplementation with vitamin C even at the moderate intake of 100mg daily.

Other investigators have reported that thiamine, riboflavin and nicotinic acid also tend to be reduced in both the intakes and the bodies of the elderly. As these three B vitamins comprise the so-called 'energy vitamins', then effects of their deficiency on the activity of older people can be imagined. Again, simple low-level supplementation with these vitamins can often change an old person's outlook on life considerably, leading to a whole new lifestyle. Vitamin B12 is also at risk, mainly because of reduced intakes of meat, poultry, fish and dairy products by the elderly.

Certain other factors make old people especially liable to mild malnutrition. They include limited mobility, loneliness and social isolation which in turn often lead to apathy, depression and impairment of appetite. The whole situation can become a vicious circle when applied particularly to the elderly disabled or to the housebound.

The obvious remedy for any ageing person is to improve the diet in terms of quality and by attempting to balance the intake of foodstuffs to ensure that all the vitamins are supplied. This, however, is easier said than done, and a simple all-round multivitamin preparation (sometimes with minerals) taken daily will at least ensure the minimum intake of vitamins without reference to those in the food. During the winter months, extra vitamin C (say 300 to 500mg daily) may also be needed to ward off infections that are prevalent at that time of the year.

Are you pregnant or breast-feeding?

It is well established that there are profound metabolic changes associated with pregnancy, some of which continue even after the mother has given birth and starts breast-feeding her child. During pregnancy the mother becomes more efficient in her utilization of both protein and energy, laying down considerable reserves during the first six months. These reserves are then drawn upon during the last three months and throughout the period when she is breast-feeding. Whilst protein and energy (in the form of fat) can be stored within the body, there is nowhere that the water-soluble vitamins can be accumulated for later use. Hence the fact that all authorities who recommend minimum daily intakes of vitamins suggest extra intakes during pregnancy and breast feeding.

The mother needs extra vitamins to ensure, first, the growth of the baby inside her and second, to supply the body, once born, with adequate vitamin reserves. The increased demand for vitamins increases whilst she is breast feeding because the suckling's needs are met only from the mother's milk. Obviously, if the mother is to meet those increased needs of nutrients (including vitamins) by eating ordinary foods then she will have to eat greater quantities. Once her needs and those of the child are reached, any excess calories will be laid down as fat and obesity may then become a problem.

The answer, to prevent excessive calorie intake whilst maintaining adequate vitamin levels, is thus to take extra of those micronutrients in the form of supplements. Many women are supplied with these by their medical practitioner but it is likely that all pregnant women will benefit from supplementation. This should be at a level sufficient to provide the extra requirements during pregnancy and breast feeding, and there is no point in taking more than is necessary. Although high intakes of vitamins have never been proved to be detrimental to the mother or to the foetus, apart perhaps from vitamin A, neither is it known with certainty if these intakes are safe. The UK authorities, for example, recommend no more than 2,250µg (7,500 i.u.) vitamin A to be taken daily as a supplement during pregnancy.

The safest regime is best worked out from the table below which indicates what various authorities suggest to the pregnant and nursing mother. At least these will ensure that no one suffers even mild deficiency.

Many studies have indicated that pregnant women are most likely to suffer from marked decreases in their blood levels of vitamin A, nicotinic acid, pyridoxine, vitamin B12 and vitamin C. To these must now be added the B vitamin folic acid. Pyridoxine is one vitamin that has been studied with reference to its requirements during pregnancy.

The existence of a pyridoxine deficiency in pregnancy has been suspected for over 30 years but the medical profession has never agreed as to the value of giving the vitamin during this period of a woman's life.

One study that attempted to resolve the problem was carried out in West Germany in 1973. Of the 458 women with uncomplicated pregnancies who were studied, between 40 and 60 percent were found to be low in vitamin B6 on all the criteria measured.

It can, therefore, be assumed that at least 50 per cent pregnant women are likely to have low blood levels of pyridoxine and presumably would benefit from supplementation. Although an improved diet may be sufficient to raise the blood levels of the vitamin to the norm, the quantities in food are not particularly high and the vitamin itself is likely to be needed. A daily intake of at least 10mg of pyridoxine has been calculated to be needed by a pregnant woman if the metabolism is to be maintained at the same level as that of a non-pregnant female of the same age. This cannot be obtained from the diet which is why the table below does not quote it.

There are other possible benefits of vitamin supplementation to a pregnant woman in addition to ensuring she is not marginally deficient. There is good evidence from various clinical trials that vitamin supplementation during pregnancy is associated with a lower than predicted incidence of the disease spina bifida in women who have already given birth to an afflicted child. No one is quite sure yet if one or more vitamins are involved in increasing the chances of spina bifida when they are deficient, but folic acid is believed to be specifically protective against the condition. Large scale trials recently reported appear to establish that folic acid may have a role in preventing spina bifida. An extra daily intake of 400µg is sufficient. Larger doses have to be prescribed. Meanwhile, it does appear to be a sensible precaution for any pregnant woman to ensure that her daily intake of all vitamins is adequate, either by carefully considering her diet or by taking a low-level all-round multivitamin preparation.

| VITAMIN | PREGNANCY | | | | | | BREAST–FEEDING | | | | | |
	AUS	CAN	NZ	UK	FAO-USA	WHO	AUS	CAN	NZ	UK	FAO-USA	WHO
VITA µg	750	900	750	750	1000	750	1200	1400	1200	750	1200	1200
VITD µg	10	5.0	10	10	10	2-5	10	5.0	10	10	10	10
VITE mg	–	7.0	13.5	–	10	–	–	8.0	13.5	–	11	–
VIT C mg	60	50	60	60	80	60	60	60	60	60	100	60
THIAMINE mg	1 .2	1 .2	1 .2	1 .0	1 .4	1 .0	1 .3	1 .5	1 .3	1.1	1 .6	1. I
RIBOFLAVIN mg	1.5	1.5	2.5	1.6	1.5	1.5	1.7	1.7	2.5	1.8	1.7	1.7
NICOTINIC ACID mg	19	15	18	18	15	16.8	22	25	21	21	18	18.2
PYRIDOXINE mg	2.6	2.0	2.5	–	2.6	–	3.3	2.6	2.5	–	2.5	–
FOLIC ACID µg	400	250	500	300	800	600	300	250	400	300	500	500
VIT B12 µg	3.0	4.0	4.0	–	4.0	5.0	2.5	3.5	4.0	–	4.0	4.5

Do you take the Contraceptive Pill?

More than 100 publications have now appeared in the medical press on the influence of oral contraceptives on the vitamin status of the women taking them. As oral contraceptives are long-term drugs – a woman can take them continually for many years – vitamin deficiencies can develop insidiously until they manifest themselves in various ways. Supplementation taken at sensible levels can help prevent deficiencies and hence reduce the chances of adverse effects.

There is good evidence that the body tissues of women taking the contraceptive pill are unsaturated with respect to vitamin C. This is reflected in higher excretion rates of the vitamin in the urine of these women compared to those levels in women using other forms of contraception. The vitamin C levels in the blood of those on the 'pill' are invariably lower than those women who are not and it is highly significant that it takes 500 mg vitamin C daily for treated women to reach the same blood levels as those who are not treated taking only 50 mg vitamin C daily. This suggests that the ingredients of the 'pill' cause increased turnover of the vitamin or perhaps may reduce the efficiency of its absorption. If you do decide to take 500mg or more of vitamin C while on the 'pill', make sure this vitamin is taken at least four hours after the 'pill' to ensure that the vitamin does not increase the absorption of the oestrogen component of the 'pill' to unacceptable levels.

Many of the B vitamins are also affected by the ingredients of the contraceptive pill and of these vitamins B6 or pyridoxine appear to be the most significant. The reason is that the depression often associated with the use of oral contraceptive appears to be a drug-related phenomenon that manifests itself through a reduction of pyridoxine blood levels. About one in twenty of women taking oral contraceptive become depressed with a characteristic pattern of lethargy, pessimism, anxiety, lack of sexual interest and a tendency to cry easily.

It now appears that this depression is due to interference by the synthetic highly potent oestrogen in the contraceptive pill with the normal chemical reactions in the brain. Normally certain brain substances are produced from the amino acid tryptophane under the influence of vitamin B6. However, 80 percent of women taking an oral contraceptive have an abnormal metabolism of tryptophane resulting in lowered production of the brain substance serotonin. This change in metabolism increases the body's requirement for pyridoxine so that more is needed than is the case in someone not taking the 'pill'.

The suggestion that the depression in the 'pill' takers is due to a deficiency of pyridoxine has been amply confirmed by trials indicating that the vitamin alone can reverse this depression. Women who developed the condition were treated with either pyridoxine or a dummy tablet and their response was assessed. Of 22 women tested, 11 had evidence of vitamin B6 deficiency in their blood and all of them lost the symptoms of depression when treated with the vitamin but not with the dummy tablets. In the 11 women who had no sign of deficiency of the vitamin in the blood; none responded to either pyridoxine or the dummy tablets. The vitamin B extra intakes needed to get over the depression induced by the contraceptive pill varied, but at least 25mg daily can be regarded as the norm.

Other B vitamins reduced by the action of the ingredients of the contraceptive pill include riboflavin, thiamine and vitamin B12. Supplementary intakes needed to restore the normal vitamin status of those women taking it have been calculated as thiamine 5mg; riboflavin 10mg; vitamin B12 4µg. Folic acid levels may be affected as well but fewer women show reduced blood levels of this vitamin. A daily supplement of 300µg should suffice to restore the body to normal. Nicotinic acid requirements from the diet may be reduced because the amino acid tryptophane is diverted to making this instead of being used in synthesis of brain substances in the absence of vitamin B6. However, as the tryptophane made within the body is normalised by vitamin B6 therapy, nicotinic acid synthesis also reaches norrnal levels and the balance between dietary and internal sources of nicotinic acid is restored.

The fat-soluble vitamin A may increase in concentration in the blood in those taking oral contraceptives, perhaps by virtue of an increase in the specific protein that binds the vitamin. This has little significance and can be ignored. What cannot be ignored is the reduced vitamin E levels in the blood that are a feature in those taking the 'pill'. As much as 200 i.u. of vitamin E daily may be required to restore normal values. There is no evidence for a reduction in vitamin D, or K, or the B vitamins pantothenic acid and biotin.

Unless the vitamin deficiencies induced by the contraceptive pill are remedied, the consequences may be serious. Typical signs of deficiency are a general malaise and depression together with increased susceptibility to infections and skin problems. These were the most common signs of deficiency found in a survey of 46,000 women who were taking the 'pill' in Britain. In addition there are several reports of adverse psychiatric, skin and blood side effects of oral contraceptives which responded to specific vitamin therapy. It has also been suggested that the prevalence of thrombosis in these women may be related to vitamin deficiency, with specific reference to vitamin E. All of these results would suggest that any woman taking the contraceptive pill should be aware of possible vitamin deficiencies which are easily overcome by simple supplementation.

Are you convalescing?

Anyone who has suffered an illness or is recovering from an operation is likely to be mildly deficient in vitamins because of a variety of factors. Illness usually gives rise to loss of appetite so the food eaten is reduced and this is parallelled by lowered vitamin intakes in the diet. In addition, the metabolism or excretion of some vitamins may be increased. A prime example is where the blood level of vitamin C drops dramatically at the commencement of an illness, particularly when the complaint is due to an infection.

If the illness is associated with the gastro-intestinal tract, as well as the possibility that normal food intakes are restricted, then the absorption of vitamins may be curtailed. This is highly significant when the condition is associated with fat malabsorption since this, in turn, will adversely affect the uptake of the fat-soluble vitamins. Vitamin A is of paramount importance in strengthening the body's resistance to infection yet many illnesses cause rapid depletion of the vitamin. Blood and tissue levels of the vitamin must, therefore, be maintained and in the absence of dietary supplies supplementation must be sought.

The deficiency of vitamins induced by the nature of the illness and a reduced food intake can be exacerbated by any medical treatment used to treat the complaint. Many drugs, as we have seen previously can have a deleterious effect upon the vitamin status of the body by preventing absorption of the essential micronutrients; by causing excessive excretion of them; by reducing their activity and neutralizing their effects. Most drugs are perhaps only used for short periods of time but they can still reduce vitamin levels sufficient to cause a mild deficiency. This in turn, of course, may slow down the rate of recovery from the illness. The rule in any period of convalescence is therefore to restore the vitamin balance of the body as quickly as possible and supplementation, combined with a good diet, is usually essential.

When the body has been damaged either by accidental injury or a surgical operation, certain vitamins are essential to speed up the healing process. Lack of vitamins C and E, for example, will slow down the rate of healing. Both vitamins should be taken before an impending operation in order to build up body levels and also during the period of con-valescence to maintain these levels. Daily intakes of 400 i.u. vitamin E and 500mg vitamin C should suffice.

The vitamin B complex will also be severely depleted during many illnesses and should be taken at moderate levels. In addition, the mineral zinc which complements the action of many vitamins is essential during the post-operation period. Zinc, amongst other functions, is needed to release vitamin A from its reserves in the liver and hence harness its power to help the body recover from medical and surgical illnesses.

Do you smoke and/or drink?

Those twin habits, smoking tobacco and drinking alcohol, have more in common than the problems encountered when they are taken in excess. They both have a deleterious effect upon the vitamin status of the body. In addition, some of these ill-effects are due to a poisonous substance called acetaldehyde which is not only present in tobacco smoke but is produced from alcohol by the body's own metabolic processes. It is not generally realised that when alcohol is drunk, only about 5 per cent of it is excreted as such in the expired air and in the urine. The rest is burned to produce energy via the ordinary metabolic cycles functioning within the body.

As acetaldehyde is the first substance produced from alcohol on this metabolic pathway, and as it is a poisonous substance, its presence in the body is usually of a transitory nature. Similarly, when taken into the blood from tobacco smoke via the lungs, acetaldehyde is normally quickly disposed of. However, the vitamins needed to burn off the acetaldehyde are those which are destroyed to the greater degree by it so when these vitamins are deficient, the ability of the body to dispose of acetaldehyde, from either source, is severely curtailed. Let us now look at those vitamins found to be affected by smoking and drinking.

There have been many reports indicating a possible association between cigarette smoking and ascorbic acid (vitamin C) deficiency. One study compared 154 non-smokers with 100 smokers and showed that plasma vitamin C decreased progressively with increased cigarette consumption. A paper in *Nutrition Today* reported evidence that smokers tended to show lowered utilization of vitamin C with less storage and higher excretion than in non-smokers. The author concluded that smokers would need twice as much vitamin C intake as non-smokers to maintain comparable blood levels. The whole relationship between smoking and vitamin C has been reviewed and the evidence available suggested there may be a good case for the preventative and possibly therapeutic use of ascorbic acid in combating some of the untoward effects of heavy smoking. The drinker of alcohol is also prone to vitamin C deficiency.

Vitamin B6 is another essential food factor that has been found to be at risk in smokers and drinkers. One study compared smoking and non-smoking human males and showed that the presence of nicotine in cigarette smoke reduced the blood levels of vitamin B6. Another study implicated the carbon monoxide of cigarette smoke in the destruction of vitamin B6 in the body leading to low levels in the blood. The blood disorders produced by alcohol have been reported in the *American Journal of Medicine* where B6 deficiency and deficiencies of other vitamins were found in the blood. There was no clear indication whether alcohol produced the deficiency by causing malabsorption of the vitamins or by causing a direct toxic action on the liver. Others have made similar observations.

Lowered blood levels of thiamine produced by drinkers of alcohol have been confirmed by many researchers who performed their studies using radioactive thiamine in their patients. They showed that alcohol interferes with vitamin B1 utilization by the liver and causes decreased absorption of the vitamin from the gastro-intestinal system.

The effect of constituents of tobacco smoke on the enzyme systems of man has also been studied and the evidence indicated that inhibitors in smoke deactivate sulphur-hydrogen groups needed in the defence mechanisms of the body and so reduce its resistance to toxic compounds. The relevance of replacement of SH compounds such as the amino acid to cysteine to restore body protection was therefore clear. Evidence is also accumulating on the effect of the mineral zinc on man's tolerance to ingested alcohol. Zinc is an essential component of the enzyme-detoxicating system for alcohol, but its levels appear to decrease with increasing intake of alcohol.

There is thus ample evidence that the inhalation of tobacco smoke and the ingestion of alcohol may put the individual at risk with reference to certain essential food constituents.

It is well established that one of the most irritating components of tobacco smoke is acetaldehyde. Drinking alcohol also causes the blood level of acetaldehyde to rise. The ill effects of acetaldehyde are seen in the recognised medical treatment of alcoholics where a drug is given deliberately to stop the further detoxification of acetaldehyde produced from alcohol. If alcohol is drunk after the drug has been taken, the ill-effects are so intense as to discourage further drinking. Under ordinary conditions of smoking and drinking the prime consideration is therefore the removal of the acetaldehyde inhaled or produced from alcohol. Nicotine is another major toxic constituent of tobacco smoke that must be removed.

Experimental evidence has indicated that a combination of vitamin C, cysteine and glucose has a better antidotal effect against nicotine and acetaldehyde than vitamin C alone. A combination of vitamin C and cysteine was found to be the best detoxicating mixture against nicotine. A combination of vitamin C, thiamine (vitamin B1) and cysteine was the best detoxicant of acetaldehyde produced by smoking and drinking. When guinea-pigs were given nicotine in tobacco smoke, vitamin C absorption was delayed and reduced. Like man, guinea-pigs rely on extraneous sources of vitamin C since neither can make it.

This means, therefore, that the very food constituents that are required for dealing with the toxic products resulting from smoking and drinking are exactly those that are likely to be deficient in individuals who smoke and/or drink. In addition there is also the possibility of low levels of vitamin B6 and zinc. To ensure that adequate quantities of these constituents are available to the smoker and the drinker they should take a vitamin C supplement (500mg); vitamin B1 (20mg); vitamin B6 (5mg); and zinc (4mg) daily. The best way to avoid a hangover is to take this combination before drinking, while drinking, and most importantly just before sleep. The detoxicating effect of the mineral and vitamins will function while asleep.

Smokers would, in addition, be advised to take beta-carotene daily at a level of 15mg. This substance has been shown in animal experiments to protect the lungs against the cancer-inducing substances in tobacco smoke. At this level, beta-carotene is harmless and can be taken on a regular basis indefinitely. Studies on its protective effect against lung and other cancers are being undertaken at present in human beings but in view of its low toxicity, it is worth a smoker taking beta-carotene regularly even though the question of its action against lung cancer in man has not yet been resolved.

Vitamin A appears to protect the body against certain cancers, including those of the lung, but it may not be as efficient as beta-carotene. In addition, there is much less chance of toxic reactions from beta-carotene than from vitamin A with its high intake required. Beta-carotene is therefore the preferred prophylactic against lung cancer induced by smoking. However, the best preventative remains not to smoke tobacco at all.

Are you slimming?

It has been estimated that some 50 per cent of people in the West are overweight. From the number of slimming regimes available and the advice given by experts (and others) it is obvious that removal of excess weight constantly occupies the thoughts of many people. Here we are talking about overweight due to over-eating. We are not concerned with white fat, brown fat, slow burners, fat burners or any of the other hypothetical concepts put forward to explain why some individuals are overweight. Nor shall we consider excessive weight due to hormonal upsets or other medical problems or medical treatment, all of which are best left to the practitioner. We shall discuss first why people who eat too much are overweight, and then consider the hazards that many encounter when embarking upon a diet eaten with the prime purpose of reducing calorie intake, but with little attention to the requirements of those other essential nutrients, vitamins and minerals.

The body requires only so much energy to function effectively each day, represented by a basic amount necessary for essential life processes, plus a variable amount that depends upon the physical activity of the individual. Even the basic requirements vary amongst people and depend upon age, sex, height, body weight, mental activity and temperament. Basic requirements decrease with age after 25 or so years, and it is the fact that these are less, but food intake remains unaltered and contributes to middle-age spread.

Food intake is energy intake because all food is capable of being converted into energy. When food that is eaten is not being converted into energy, it is stored within the body to be used at some later date. The storage of energy within the body is achieved in the main by the laying down of fat. Some is stored as animal starch or glycogen, particularly in the liver and muscles, but this should be regarded as first-line reserves and is of no consequence in producing a condition of overweight.

Fat storage, of course, has other functions. It serves to act as an insulator against the cold and it is deposited around essential internal organs such as the kidney where it acts as a protective barrier. Fat is also nature's way of saving energy 'for a rainy day'. The conservation of energy as fat is of prime importance to wild animals as they have to eat when they can and have no guarantee of regular meals. They are able to live off their fat reserves until the next feed, which can be hours or, more likely, days away. Most human beings have no such problems. Their three meals a day are virtually guaranteed and too often food intake is geared to appetite rather than to necessity. Small wonder then that energy intake exceeds energy output, with the result that the difference is laid down as body fat. We are laying down reserves of energy with little chance of ever using them. Body weight must increase under these circumstances.

It is important to realise that the three food constituents, carbohydrate, fat and protein, can all be converted by the body into fat. Many diets use the high protein concept where carbohydrate and fat intake are curtailed but lots of protein is eaten. This is fine up to a point but it must be remembered that gram for gram protein supplies 4.00 calories compared to 3.75 calories for carbohydrate. Excess protein is just as liable to be laid down as fat as are starch and sugars. Fat of course, contributes the higher energy at 9 calories per gram, but don't forget alcohol at 7 calories per gram. Hence the ideal diet is balanced in these three basic food constituents but if this intake is reduced, other problems are introduced which are concerned with those essential food constituents, vitamins and minerals.

Foods vary tremendously in their content of vitamins and minerals; this is why only a balanced, good quality and varied diet will supply all the essential nutrients for health. Most vitamins are sensitive chemical compounds which means that any excess cooking or bad storage of foods can often destroy them irreversibly. Minerals cannot be destroyed but they can be removed from foods by over-refining and processing; they are often discarded in water used for cooking, and they are liable to be irreversibly bound to other food constituents, making them unavailable to the body. Minerals in our food must ultimately come from the soil, yet it is known that this varies widely in its mineral content and is often lacking in essential trace elements. It is hoped that a normal intake of food taken from a wide variety of sources and cooked expertly will supply all the necessary vitamins and minerals. How then can someone on a slimming diet with a restricted food intake hope to obtain their full requirements of these nutrients? The answer is that they are unlikely to. In fact, slimmers are now recognized officially as a group of the population who may be liable to vitamin and mineral deficiency when their slimming regimes are undertaken without professional advice.

Just how deficient in vitamins and minerals could an individual on a slimming diet be? If we take an average calorie requirement from a normal diet for an adult female to be say, 2,300 calories and an adult male to need 2,900 calories, we can assume that the amount of food to supply this would also supply the daily requirements of vitamins and minerals. When these people reduce their intake of food energy to the conventional 1,000 calories there must also be a concomitant decrease in their intake of the essential nutrients. Unfortunately, however, the body requirements for vitamins and minerals are the same regardless of the calorie intake. The only exception to this is thiamine or vitamin B1 whose requirements are related to carbohydrate intake; the more carbohydrate eaten the more vitamin B1 is needed. All other vitamins are necessary for health in minimum quantities that have no relationship to energy intake.

Individual items of food have varying contents of the various vitamins and minerals and there is a risk that in avoiding some high calorie foods when on a slimming diet there is a greater risk of deficiency, in particular vitamins and minerals. Potatoes, for example, are our main source of vitamin C, not because they are the richest source of the vitamin but due essentially to the large bulk eaten. Unfortunately, potatoes are also usually the first item of food that a slimmer will remove from the diet since they are an excellent source of calories. The slimmer should therefore look to low calorie alternatives rich in vitamin C such as unsweetened natural fruit juice and raw fruit and lightly-cooked green vegetables.

Cereals are rich in the vitamin B complex yet slimmers tend to avoid these foods because of their high carbohydrate content. Bread is an important source of the vitamin B group and is another example of a food usually taken in large quantity that contributes a large proportion of these vitamins to the body.

Where then are the slimmers, who usually cut down on bread, going to obtain their B vitamins? Most meats and particularly liver are very rich in the B vitamins, so this presents no problem to the meat eater. However, the vegetarian can look to a variety of foods. Fortunately, whole raw nuts are a rich source of all these vitamins (apart from vitamin B12) and remember that each ounce will contribute a good share of the daily protein requirements. Eggs, of course, are a complete food that should feature in any slimmer's diet. Dried fruit will also yield useful amounts of the B group without making too large a hole in the calorie count. Green vegetables are also useful sources but it is important not to destroy the vitamins by overcooking.

It is unlikely that these vegetable foods will give you sufficient vitamin B12 and it is essential to ensure some intake of meats or dairy products on a slimming diet to ensure adequate amounts of this vitamin. The liver carries useful stores of vitamin B12 in most individuals but on any long-term slimming regime these could be depleted if the intake of meat and dairy products is curtailed. Most dairy products are avoided by slimmers because of their high fat content so it is important to make sure of one's vitamin B12 requirements by taking some meat.

Vegetarians may wish to obtain their B12 from cheeses at the expense of their calorie intake but a supplement is the safest and easiest way to ensure their B12 requirements.

Folic acid is unlikely to present a problem to the slimmer as the richest sources are green leaf vegetables and salads – both are foods that tend to be eaten in large quantity on a calorie-restricted diet. Liver, which should also feature in a slimmer's diet, is high in folic acid and has the advantage of being rich in the type of folic acid that can be used by man.

The vitamins most at risk in slimmers are the fat soluble A, D and E. This is because by their very nature they are associated with fats and oils that the slimmer tends to avoid. During winter months the food is the more important source of vitamin D and is found in dairy products, fish and liver. A low intake of these will reflect in low body levels of the vitamin. In the absence of dairy products a daily supplement is advisable. There should however be no problem in the summer as long as sufficient sunlight is allowed to fall on the skin, since the action of ultra-violet rays actually produces vitamin D in the skin. Switching from full cream milk to the skimmed variety will also deprive the slimmer of the fat soluble vitamins which must then be obtained from other sources.

The meat eater should derive ample vitamin A from liver as long as this is taken as part of the diet. Fish is also an excellent source of both vitamins A and D. The vegetarian will, it is hoped, obtain his or her vitamin A from carotenes that are found in plants, but remember that not all carotene are precursors of the vitamin. Carrots, spinach, broccoli and Brussels sprout are particularly rich in carotene that will give rise to vitamin A.

Vitamin E occurs in the highest concentration in vegetable oils and, although the slimmer may be wary of these in view of their high calorie content, some should feature in every diet. In addition, these oils supply the essential polyunsaturated fatty acids that are needed in many body functions. A daily intake of oils will therefore ensure adequate vitamin E and vitamin F (another name for polyunsaturated fatty acids). Vitamin E is widely distributed in many foods but its concentration is low and when the actual quantity of food consumed is reduced as in the slimmer, a low intake of vitamin E follows. The simplest way to take vitamin E is in capsules that contribute not only the vitamin but also the polyunsaturated fatty acids. The calorific value of these capsules is so low as to be negligible.

Meat and fish are generally regarded as suitable for slimmers and fortunately these foods are good sources of many of the vitamins mentioned. However, for a variety of reasons such foods are not always eaten by the slimmer in sufficient quantity to yield the full complement of vitamins necessary. In addition, meat and fish are usually low in vitamins C and E, both of which are required in the highest quantities amongst the vitamins. Therefore, a balanced diet should be sought to incorporate other foods rich in these vitamins. Even so, on a daily intake of 1,000 calories there is the possibility of mild deficiency. Vegetarian slimmers are most likely to obtain a balanced vitamin intake but this is tempered by a lower bulk of food than is usual and their total intake is likely to be less.

The simplest insurance for anyone undergoing a slimming regime is a daily supplement of all the vitamins necessary to sustain life. Choose any one of the many multivitamin preparations available, any one of which per day will give sufficient vitamins without reference to those taken in the diet. We know that vitamins are essential in the processes of burning food to give energy, in the interconversion of foods and to burn off that unsightly fat that is the aim of every slimmer. A deficiency of vitamins must reflect in a less efficient system for disposing of excess weight. Minerals are just as important to health as vitamins and they act together with vitamins in controlling the metabolism of the body. We rely upon food as a source of minerals so that these too may be prone to deficiency as the amount of food eaten is reduced during slimming bouts. The minerals required in relatively large amounts such as calcium and phosphorus are present in high concentration in dairy products but these foods are often ignored by the slimmer. Shellfish contribute reasonable amounts of calcium and phosphorus but they would not be acceptable to the vegetarian. Bread and cereals are good sources of calcium but these too are foods generally avoided by slimmers. Vegetables must therefore be the most important source of calcium and phosphorus to the slimmer. Our skeleton acts as a rich reservoir of calcium but during prolonged periods of slimming the withdrawal of calcium and phosphorus from bone could tend to weaken it. In the absence of dairy products, then, a supplement of calcium must be sought.

Magnesium is widely distributed in all foods but the reduction of calories to 1,000 or so per day must adversely affect the intake of this mineral. Low magnesium in the body leads to irritability, depression, mild mental problems and muscular weakness. How often are these conditions associated with the slimmer! Magnesium is best taken as a supplement in the form of dolomite tablets. These supply calcium as well and the two minerals are in the same ratio in dolomite as in the required intake from food. They are calorie-free and dissolve in stomach acid to ensure good absorption.

Even on normal diets supplying the average calorie requirement, iron is often at risk in view of its poor absorption. The possibility of deficiency must therefore increase on a reduced calorie intake. Again the meat eater has some advantage over his or her vegetarian counterpart because the iron from meat is better absorbed than that from vegetables. Under normal circumstances this does not matter because the vegetarian makes up in quantity of vegetable foods what they lack in quality, but a reduction in food intake will almost certainly give rise to iron deficiency. In the female of child-bearing age this deficiency may be exacerbated by menstrual loss of iron and the chances of full replacement on a slimming diet are remote. Therefore, the slimmer must choose foods with a high iron content – usually of animal origin – but failing this they should seek a supplement. Iron from iron salts is notoriously difficult to absorb so that the quantity of salts taken are far in excess of that needed. Iron amino acid chelates are the nearest equivalent to the iron presented in meat (although of vegetable origin) with the result that absorption is superior to that of iron salts.

Zinc is another mineral assuming more and more importance as research continues and it tends to be associated with high protein foods. Hence, any slimming diet that is low in protein-rich constituents will be deficient in zinc.

There is considerable doubt as to whether conventional diets provide sufficient zinc so the chances of deficiency from a calorie-reduced diet are enhanced. Sea foods are particularly rich in zinc and they contribute other minerals from the sea as well as protein at the expense of a few calories. Nuts are also good sources of zinc so that the non-fish eater can obtain some of their requirements from these.

The simplest way to ensure a good intake of trace minerals daily, particularly whilst slimming, is to take kelp. Kelp is dried seaweed that has concentrated in it all of the minerals of the sea, probably the richest source of minerals of any area in the world. In addition, kelp is an excellent source of iodine which has a very important role in the body. Iodine is a constituent of thyroxine, the hormone from the thyroid gland that controls body metabolism. Low iodine levels mean a sluggish metabolism which is the last condition a slimmer would want. By ensuring an adequate iodine intake, a slimmer can make certain that the body has every chance to metabolise its food and, more importantly, turn excess fat into energy. In addition, the other minerals in kelp are essential ingredients in the enzymes necessary for the metabolic conversion of food and fat into energy.

There is little doubt that people will continue to undertake slimming diets without medical supervision for a long time to come. As long as they are aware of the need for the following they should come to no harm:

1. A minimum intake of calories, usually 800-1000 daily
2. A minimum intake of protein, usually 40-60 gram daily
3. A supplemental intake of all vitamins and minerals.

At least it is possible to ensure an adequate supply of vitamins and minerals using supplements that yield only a negligible quantity of calories. Supplementation removes some of the problems associated with dieting. All that is left then is an awareness of protein intake and the pleasure of calorie-counting.

Do you fall into one of these other categories?

THOSE UNDER STRESS

Some years ago animal experiments indicated that during periods of stress the requirements for the vitamin B complex and vitamin C increased. In any animal, under stress conditions, the body reacts by producing hormones from the glands that enable it to overcome the effects of that stress. Vitamins B and C and certain minerals are essential in the production of these hormones and so they contribute to the animal's defence against stress. A similar situation was observed in the American astronauts. During the early space flights it was discovered that although the men appeared to have adequate intakes of all the vitamins in their food, they were not sufficient for the great physical and mental stress that the astronauts underwent. On return to Earth, their blood levels of vitamins were dangerously low.

Particularly susceptible were vitamin B and C, but also vitamin E. In fact, vitamin E levels were so low that all of the astronauts developed anaemia whilst on the flight, due mainly to massive haemolysis (breakdown) of red blood cells. In later flights all the vitamin intakes were increased and the biochemical problems did not arise. Not many of us will undergo space flights but what was learned from these pioneers may help us in overcoming the stress of life.

MENSTRUATING WOMEN

We have seen that women who take the contraceptive pill are inducing in themselves an increased requirement for vitamin B6. This is due to a direct action of the synthetic female sex hormones in the preparation, but mainly the oestrogenic component, that cause increased usage of vitamin B6 and probably also reduce its absorption from the food.

A similar phenomenon is seen in some women who are not taking the contraceptive pill but still suffer the same sort of symptoms, known as Premenstrual Syndrome (PMS), ten days or so before their period is due to start. It is likely that over-production of oestrogens or reduced synthesis of the other sex hormone progesterone by the female is the prime cause of PMS. Treatment is therefore aimed at overcoming any vitamin deficiency that contributes to the hormone imbalance.

Vitamin B6 helps some women who suffer from premenstrual tension. In a trial carried out at St. Thomas's Hospital in London, vitamin B6 supplementation was compared to hormone treatment over a period of seven months. Significant improvement was seen in those treated with hormones in terms of premenstrual irritability, depression and swelling of the abdomen. An overall improvement in 73 per cent of these patients was noted with this treatment. A comparable group of women was given vitamin B6 in 100mg dose daily. At this level there was an overall improvement of symptoms in 63 per cent of the women. The results suggest that perhaps vitamin B6 should be the primary treatment of premenstrual tension as it is successful, natural, and lacks side-effects at this dose.

Simple supplementation with vitamin B6 will help many women suffering from PMS but there are always some who will not respond or whose symptoms are only partially relieved by the vitamin. In these cases another natural approach is often recommended which is not strictly replacing a vitamin deficiency but nevertheless has a vitamin-like action.

At one time the polyunsaturated fatty acids (also known as essential fatty acids) were known as vitamin F but as their mode of action became clearer it was realised that the most important member was *linoleic acid*. The designation vitamin F for this acid was eventually discarded as, although it was essential and could be obtained only from the food, its daily requirements were too high to define it as a true vitamin. Nevertheless, the term vitamin F still persists in some parts of the world.

Linoleic acid has many functions within the body, but the one that concerns us here is that of being the starting material in the production of prostaglandins. These are important hormones that control many of the essential life processes and they are produced only in the body from dietary linoleic acid. To be made into prostaglandins, linoleic acid must first be converted to gamma linoleic acid and this step appears to be the main stumbling block in conditions where prostaglandin synthesis is curtailed. For example, women who suffer PMS appear, first, to have a polyunsaturated fatty acid deficiency and, second, to be unable to produce enough gamma linoleic acid to satisfy their needs. Treatment of PMS is therefore aimed at supplying both polyunsaturated fatty acids (particularly linoleic) and gamma linoleic acid.

Oil of evening primrose is obtained from the seeds of that plant and it is one of the richer sources of both polyunsaturated fatty acids and of gamma linoleic acid. Hence, by taking the oil (usually in capsule form) for the ten days or so before a period is due, a female can ensure she has adequate intakes of linoleic and gamma linoleic acids. If her PMS is due to lack of these, supplementation with the acids will relieve her symptoms. This has been amply proved in many clinical trials.

Hence any female who suffers PMS can take vitamin B6 and/or oil of evening primrose as a perfectly natural treatment for her symptoms. This represents a self-help natural alternative to the hormone treatment prescribed by her medical practitioner and is one devoid of possible side-effects.

ASIAN IMMIGRANTS

Members of some immigrant populations often avoid certain foods for religious reasons and so create an imbalance in their nutritional intake.

Concerns have been expressed in recent years over the re-appearance of rickets due to vitamin D deficiency among Asian immigrants in the UK. The disorder is due to inadequate intake of vitamin D, plus failure in the formation of the vitamins from 7-dehydrocholesterol in the skin thanks to a lack of sunlight and the presence of pigmentation.

The obvious remedy is supplementary vitamin D in the diet, and a Government study group has decided that this is the best way to overcome deficiency. However, many Asians are vegetarians, so that good sources like cod liver oil and liver are not acceptable. They can however seek other sources such as those from irradiated yeast. Nonetheless, simply giving extra vitamin D may not be the complete answer. The recent study of white children in the UK, quoted earlier provided evidence that those who had a seaside holiday during the previous summer had a higher blood level of vitamin D during the winter than those who had not. In both children and adults, vitamin supplementation increased blood levels, but not up to the level of those exposed to sunshine all those months previously.

The answer may, therefore, be a change in diet that supplies vitamin D; supplementation in the winter months, and a more prolonged exposure to sunshine when this is available.

THOSE WHO LIVE ALONE

Another group of the population at risk from vitamin and mineral deficiencies is that consisting of those living alone. These people are often elderly and hence suffer from the same dietary problems as those mentioned previously. In addition, however, loss of a partner often induces a reluctance to cook food for one so that cheap, refined carbohydrates and simple beverages are relied upon as a staple diet. Often these people will rely upon institutional or supplied meals (in which excessive vitamin and mineral loss may be prevalent) for their dietary needs. An official study which was undertaken in 1972 found that men living alone had lower intakes of food and hence essential nutrients than those living with a wife or family.

Even younger people are not immune as they will often rely upon quick and easy-to-cook convenience foods that are not always guaranteed full nutritional value. Students fall into this category as pointed out in an official comprehensive study carried out in 1974. Intakes of vitamin C, B1 and B2 varied tremendously amongst students and the contributing factors were believed to be reliance on institutional meals, poor self catering and financial inability to purchase a good all-round nutritious diet.

Supplementation with a good all-round multivitamin preparation, whilst not replacing an improved diet, will at least ensure the minimum daily requirement of vitamins without reference to those in the food.

CHILDREN

Children are notorious as faddy eaters and nothing is more calculated to put a child off healthy nutrition than telling them that food 'is good for them'. Children often do not eat the right foods because they do not like them and instead prefer to fill up on sweet or savoury snacks that add calories but little else. Unfortunately, lack of vitamins and/or minerals during the growing period can adversely affect growth and development, both mental and physical. Medical studies on children in poor communities in the Middle East indicated that a lack of zinc was a direct cause of reduced sexual, physical and mental development. Adding extra zinc to the diet normalised their complete development. Similarly, lack of vitamin E in the diet of children can retard growth and induce anaemia, conditions that were only cured by supplementing the diet with vitamin E.

ATHLETES

Athletes in general have a greater energy requirement due to their physical exertions, but it is important for them to ensure an adequate vitamin and mineral intake to parallel those extra dietary calories. Too often the additional food an athlete takes during training or competition consists of glucose sweets and drinks and pure protein which are calories devoid of minerals and vitamins. Many sportsmen obtain at least part of their dietary intake from institutional sources like colleges, works or office restaurants, with the danger that such overcooked foods may be deficient in vitamins, particularly vitamin C. This vitamin is important in the production of body hormones which are required in higher concentration during excessive physical activity. The vitamin B complex which is concerned in the conversion of food into energy may wisely be taken during intense physical activity. Both vitamins B1 and B2 appear to be essential in recovery from fatigue. Excessive perspiration during athletic pursuits leads to loss of minerals in the sweat that can only be replaced in the food.

Blood supply to muscles must be efficient to ensure they receive a constant supply of oxygen, glucose and other nutrients. In addition, of course, the blood from the muscles must also be adequate to take away the waste products of muscle metabolism, many of which can be toxic if allowed to build up. For this reason, many athletes take extra vitamin E, up to 1,000 i.u. daily, to ensure that the supply in the blood is sufficient. The vitamin not only increases the efficiency of oxygen carriage in the blood and its uptake by the muscles but dilates the blood vessels to ensure adequate blood reaches the muscles.

HOW TO COPE?

The important question now arises: How can we overcome these deficiencies?

It would be irresponsible to say, 'Take vitamins, and don't bother about what you eat, drink or smoke'. Eating meals of natural foods that haven't been processed, refined or over-cooked must remain the basis of your vitamin supply. Reducing the amount of alcohol you drink is beneficial to general health. Stopping smoking is probably the most valuable single step towards improved health you can make.

Having said that, there remain all those situations where good eating habits are sabotaged by circumstances, whether of choice — such as slimming — or not, such as being tied to the food served in a hospital, school company canteen or other institutional catering.

In such circumstances, it is very difficult for the individual to work out where his vitamin intake may be lacking. So the best insurance against nutritional deficiencies is a daily multivitamin preparation, and it must be one rich enough in the vitamins to guarantee an adequate intake for anyone, regardless of their dietary sources. If you drink or smoke or are on 'the pill', no multivitamin preparation is sufficiently potent in individual vitamins to overcome their effects. Specific supplements for these conditions must be sought, although it must be realised that these can only help offset such effects as may be related to vitamin deficiencies caused by these drugs. There is no supplement that can protect you from their other, far-reaching effects on the body.

Finally, if you are on any long-term drug treatment, your doctor should be aware of potential vitamin deficiencies. However, these are very specialised and usually pose no problem with short term medicines. Perhaps we can change a popular quote by saying 'a multivitamin a day', rather than 'an apple a day', is more likely to keep the doctor away.

OTHER BOOKS FROM AMBERWOOD PUBLISHING ARE:

Aromatherapy – A Guide for Home Use by Christine Westwood. All you need to know about essential oils and using them. £1.99.

Aromatherapy – For Stress Management by Christine Westwood. Covering the use of essential oils for everyday stress-related problems. £2.99.

Aromatherapy – For Healthy Legs and Feet by Christine Westwood. A comprehensive guide to the use of essential oils for the treatment of legs and feet, including illustrated massage instructions. £2.99.

Aromatherapy – Simply For You by Marion Del Gaudio Mak. A clear, simple and comprehensive guide to Aromatherapy for beginners. £1.99.

Plant Medicine – A Guide for Home Use by Charlotte Mitchell MNIMH. A guide to home use giving an insight into the wonderful healing qualities of plants. £2.99.

Woman Medicine – Vitex Agnus Castus by Simon Mills MA, FNIMH. The wonderful story of the herb that has been used for centuries in the treatment of women's problems. £2.99.

Ancient Medicine – Ginkgo Biloba by Dr Desmond Corrigan BSc(Pharms), MA, Phd, FLS, FPSI. Improved memory, circulation and concentration are associated in this book with medicine from this fascinating tree. £2.99.

Indian Medicine – The Immune System by Desmond Corrigan BSc(Pharms), MA, Phd, FLS, FPSI. An intriguing account of the history and science of the plant called Echinacea and its power to influence the immune system. £2.99.

Herbal First Aid by Andrew Chevallier BA, MNIMH. A beautifully clear reference book of natural remedies and general first aid in the home. £2.99.

Natural Taste – Herbal Teas, A Guide for Home Use by Andrew Chevallier BA, MNIMH. This beautifully illustrated book containing a comprehensive compendium of Herbal Teas gives information on how to make it, its benefits, history and folklore. £2.99.

Signs & Symptoms of Vitamin Deficiency by Dr Leonard Mervyn BSc, PhD, C.Chem, FRCS. A home guide for self diagnosis which explains and assesses Vitamin Therapy for the prevention of a wide variety of diseases and illnesses. £2.99.

Eyecare Eyewear – For Better Vision by Mark Rossi Bsc, MBCO. A complete guide to eyecare and eyewear including an assessment of the types of spectacles and contact lenses available and the latest corrective surgical procedures. £3.99.